Normal
People Do
the Craziest
Things

Dr. David Hawkins

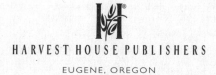

HARVEST HOUSE PUBLISHERS

EUGENE, OREGON

This book contains stories in which the author has changed some people's names and some details of their situations to protect their privacy.

Cover photo © Comstock Images / Jupiterimages Unlimited.

Cover by Koechel Peterson & Associates, Inc., Minneapolis, Minnesota

NORMAL PEOPLE DO THE CRAZIEST THINGS
Copyright © 2009 by David Hawkins
Published by Harvest House Publishers
Eugene, Oregon 97402
www.harvesthousepublishers.com

Library of Congress Cataloging-in-Publication Data

Hawkins, David, 1951-
Normal people do the craziest things / David Hawkins.
    p. cm.
Includes bibliographical references.
ISBN 978-0-7369-2478-8 (pbk.)
1. Mental health—Religious aspects—Christianity. 2. Self-acceptance—Religious aspects—Christianity. I. Title.
BT732.4.H38 2009
248.8'6—dc22

                                                                    2008049428

Printed in the United States of America

09 10 11 12 13 14 15 16 17 / BP-NI / 10 9 8 7 6 5 4 3 2 1

This book is dedicated lovingly to my grandson,
Caleb Joshua Hawkins,
who is just beginning to find his place in this world.

You have already made a delightful
impact on many lives, Caleb,
including mine.

Acknowledgments

The galley of this book came in the mail just a few weeks ago—another milestone in its publishing journey. If the galleys are here, the finished product can't be far off.

A book comes to life in many stages. It begins with an idea, and Terry Glaspey at Harvest House Publishers, my dear friend, is to thank for embracing the idea and nudging it through the publisher's committee. Thanks again, Terry for championing my "crazy" ideas.

I dedicated many weekends to writing this book, and I thank my wife, Christie, for unselfishly giving me the time, space, and nurture to complete the project. Christie is also my first-line editor. This isn't always an easy relationship as she cuts out some of my precious words. Her choices, however, have always made the writing better. Thanks, Christie, for your encouragement and for making my writing tighter, stronger, and brighter.

After being trimmed down to fighting weight, the book goes to Gene Skinner, Harvest House editor par excellence, who has edited many of my books. (How many is it now, Gene?) When the book reaches Gene's desk, I know I'm in for another round of work. It's all for the best, as Gene makes suggestions and requests that make for a better book. You improve my books, Gene, in ways I'll never know. Thanks for being such an insightful, gifted editor and good friend.

Ready to go out the publishing door, the book becomes dependent on the gifted hands of the professional marketing and sales teams at Harvest House Publishers. You are so easy to work with, and I've grown to appreciate and enjoy each of you so very much. Thank you for believing in me and my writing as we work together in encouraging people.

Finally, praise God from whom all blessings flow.

Contents

Prologue: We're Not as Crazy as We Think   7

1. Crazy, Normal, or Something In Between? 17

2. Everyone Looks So Normal 33

3. Courageously Exploring Inner Space 51

4. You Really Want to Be Normal? 71

5. We're All a Little Bit Nuts 87

6. Everybody's Talkin' About Me 105

7. Emotional Myopia 123

8. If You Only Knew 143

9. But My Family *Is* Certifiably Nuts 159

10. Overwhelmed, Under Slept, and a Little Bit Tense 175

11. Dance of the Porcupines 191

12. Now You See Me, Now You Don't 209

Epilogue: Perfectly You 225

Notes 235

Prologue: We're Not as Crazy as We Think

Has the fact that you're completely psycho managed to escape your attention?

BIANCA STRATFORD
IN *TEN THINGS I HATE ABOUT YOU*

We're all a little bit nuts.

OK, I hope we've got that settled.

Yes, we're all a little bit nuts, but thankfully, we're not as crazy as we think.

What if, after you tell me that you're afraid of heights, you count to ten before stepping off the curb, and you *really* dislike your mother-in-law, I still proclaimed you to be normal? What if, after hearing you've been divorced twice, you are struggling in your current marriage, and you have a horrific temper no one but your mate has seen, I still insisted you're not as crazy as you think?

If I could prove to you that you are normal, would you be interested in reading this book? If I shared with you what I've discovered from thousands of hours consulting with clients—young and old, short and tall, small and large, rich and poor—and authoritatively declared that you were quite normal, would you breathe a sigh of relief?

I listen to people's secrets for a living. After 34 years of counseling, I've heard it all. Jerry Springer has nothing on me. I listen with rarely even a hint of surprise as people tell me about their foibles, mishaps, quirks, and unusual characteristics—and I share with them that I've heard it all before. They're not as crazy as they think. In fact, more often than not, they are normal.

You can imagine the relief people feel when I share this news. We all have an underlying fear that we're somehow different, inferior, or perhaps worse—mentally ill or crazy.

Most of us have lain awake at night obsessing about questions like these:

- Do others worry as much as I do?
- Are my fears normal, or are they over the edge?
- Are my fears and anxieties considered mental illness?
- Do others have these kinds of moods?
- Are other families as dysfunctional, loud, obnoxious, hysterical, deceptive, dishonest, or crazy as mine?
- Do other people need to talk about their concerns as much as I do?
- If other people knew what I was thinking, would they think I'm crazy?

Alone with this racket, our thoughts swirl in our mind, and we often end up thinking the worst. We know the truth about ourselves. Or at least we think we do!

A 25-year-old woman compulsively twists her hair. She is vaguely aware she does it and wishes she could simply stop—but she can't. Feeling self-conscious when she catches herself, she wonders what is making her so anxious. But when we step back and take another look, this behavior isn't so odd. In fact, it's quite normal and very common.

A 35-year-old woman doesn't let her preadolescent children spend time alone in the mall, fearing they'll be kidnapped. Her children are self-confident and able to take care of themselves. Somewhere deep inside she knows her fears are largely irrational. But who hasn't been protective of their children, worrying about their safety? This behavior too is very normal.

A 40-year-old man has temper tantrums, screaming at his employees and family over trivial matters. He hates his irritability but can't seem to let go of these minor issues. Deep inside, he knows that his anger is irrational. He alone knows that he cares about people and that his anger is not the totality of his character.

A 50-year-old woman wants to lose weight and has tried every possible diet. She envies skinny women on the covers of magazines at checkout counters. She wishes they were fat and ugly, and then she feels guilty for having such thoughts.

These people are like you and me. They wonder and worry about themselves, just as you and I wonder and worry about ourselves. Without the benefit of feedback from others, however, they make faulty conclusions like these:

- I really am a nutcase.
- I really do have more worries and fears than others.
- My problems have jumped into the category of mental illness.
- My family is certifiably nuts.
- I don't want others to know what I'm thinking.
- I better keep these thoughts and feelings to myself.

Our worries and fears wander around in our heads like orphans without a home. They are unattached and unappreciated. This must change. We're going to make friends with these fears and behaviors. We're going to give them an understanding and welcoming home—a home based squarely in reality.

Reality

In reality, we are all a little bit nuts. We've all got goofy fears and quirks that make up our individuality. If only we could see ourselves that way.

Instead of feeling bad about our quirks and problems, wouldn't it be great if we could realize they are simply aspects of our nature that make us who we are? Wouldn't it be wonderful to stop feeling ashamed or embarrassed about them and begin to truly believe that these traits are what make us human?

Notice the popularity of television shows like *The Oprah Winfrey Show, Dr. Phil,* and other talk shows. These programs are hugely popular because they allow us to peek into the lives of others. We hope that they struggle with some of the same fears and oddities we do. We smile at their adversities—not because we want them to suffer, but because their challenges are our challenges.

Sometimes we even laugh. This stuff isn't staged! These people really do have the same insecurities we have! They really do fight with their mate, pout when they're angry, and stuff their feelings when they're upset. Maybe we're not so different from one another after all.

Group Therapy

Imagine with me one gigantic group therapy session, with God as our therapist. In this fantasy, everyone in the world sits in a humongous circle, holding hands. Frightened fat people stand next to compulsively thin people, insecure rich people stand next to insecure poor people, and old, long-haired hippies stand next to tattooed young people. For the sake of my fantasy, God is 65 years old, tanned, dressed in khakis, and sporting a short, white goatee. He has a gentle, welcoming smile. In a deep, warm voice, he shares a few words.

"I'm glad you all agreed to join my group. This group therapy is for everyone with any kind of hang-up, and as you can clearly see, that includes everyone. I want to reassure you that no problems are worse than others. Your quirk or addiction or personality trait is no more troublesome than anyone else's. The differences you see are only skin deep because inside, you're all alike. You're all just a little bit crazy, and that's just fine. So you can relax."

With that, God asks who would like to begin talking about his or her life. The secrecy and feelings of inferiority fade as we all share our story and gradually realize just how much alike we are.

We obviously cannot create a literal world community, but this book offers you a unique opportunity to engage in a kind of group therapy. It provides many of the benefits of group therapy, including a chance to check out other people's lives and compare yourself to them. In the safety of your home, you can find out whether your reality is really all that different from others'.

Support groups are fantastic. I started a men's group at my church that met every week for seven years, and I never missed except for vacations, births, deaths, and catastrophic illnesses.

That group fluctuated from five to seven men. I shared my problems and my darkest secrets. I shared embarrassing feelings, thoughts, and actions. At first I shared cautiously, worrying these guys would think I was crazy. As time went on, and after feeling safe, I shared practically anything without as much as a raised eyebrow.

I shared about feeling exhausted from excessive work but feeling as if I should be able to keep up with others who worked longer hours than I did. I shared my feelings of anxiety, which came with the exhaustion. I shared fears that my life would spin out of control. I shared about the conflict I had with my wife over my long hours of work and the guilt I felt for missing many important events in my children's lives. I shared, listened, and shared some more. As the men listened to my dark secrets, I received an odd reaction.

"Yeah? So what?" these guys would ask when I shared something I thought would freak them out.

"I know what you mean," they would say almost casually.

"Yeah, I did that too," another would add, referring to the neglect of his children.

"I'm having a hard time in my marriage too," another added. "I want to be a good husband, but it's tough."

I couldn't shock these men. Usually, someone else had experienced what I had experienced. Someone had felt what I had felt. Someone had done what I had done.

Gradually my feelings changed. I began to feel normal. If my thoughts weren't strange, if my actions weren't weird or bizarre, and if my feelings were similar to feelings these men had, then evidently I wasn't as crazy as I thought. The relief I felt from this support was incredible. It was lifesaving.

This book isn't a worldwide support group, but it can provide many of the benefits of your own support group:

You'll connect emotionally with others. Throughout the pages of this book, you'll read stories of people who thought they were odd. You'll discover from this emotional connection that you can understand your problems and deal with them effectively.

You'll lose your sense of isolation from keeping your problems a secret. You'll discover you're not in this thing alone. Your problems are like other people's problems, and theirs have similarities to yours. We truly are all in this together.

You'll learn more about your particular problem. We'll talk about common emotional problems and help you see that your experience is normal. You'll become more informed and less likely to pathologize your problems. With the right information, you can put issues in perspective.

You'll release pent-up emotions. When you get your concerns out on the table and realize they are not as hideous as you might think, you'll sigh with relief and feel freer to experience and express other emotions.

Finally, you'll discover that God made you to be the unique person you are. He didn't make any mistakes when He created you. Your life story was in His mind at the foundation of the world. When we discover that He is holding our lives safely in His hands, we can fully lean into the powerful truth that we're not as crazy as we think.

These are invaluable experiences to take away from our group therapy experience. What a relief to feel normal! By the time you finish this book, you'll no longer feel as if you're on the wrong side of the fence. You'll see that you're part of one really big family.

What If I Am Crazy?

You may doubt that your story is like anyone else's. You've felt different your entire life, and no book can change your mind, right? Wrong. You're going to see that your experiences all fit within the realm of normalcy. Even if your experiences are extreme, you'll see that others have felt the way you feel, they have thought the way you think, and they have done many of the things you've done.

However, changing old patterns of thinking will take effort. Anyone who joins a group or goes to counseling has to be willing to ask some tough questions. People who are willing to sit in front of others and reveal the inner workings of their minds must be willing to receive feedback that might not be complimentary.

I applaud you for picking up this book and joining our group. We need you. We need more people who are willing to admit they don't have it all together and who will talk about some of the quirky things they think and do.

One of my favorite authors is Susan Ariel Rainbow Kennedy, otherwise known as SARK. She has written a lot of books, including *The Bodacious Book of Succulence*. As you can probably imagine from her name and the title of her book, she's a self-avowed misfit. She's a nonconforming, radical, creative sort. She won't be pigeonholed into any category. She openly admits she doesn't have it all together. She lives out what I'm talking about—we're all a little bit nuts, and saying that out loud is OK. In fact, living it out loud is OK.

Perhaps you picked up this book because the title made you smile, or maybe you're looking for reassurance that you really are OK, or you might be looking for answers to certain problems or situations. We all have hidden thoughts and behaviors. But if you're willing to live out loud and let others see what's going on inside, then good for you!

SARK didn't get to her place of self-acceptance overnight, so be careful about being in a hurry. You may not quite be ready to give up your fears of being different. Don't worry—it will happen.

Simply picking up this book is a big step. You won't be disappointed.

Holding your thoughts out where you can review them lovingly but objectively is a huge step. I'm confident you'll discover that your problems are somewhat similar to mine, but you may find that some areas of your life really are different from mine. That's to be expected. Can you take a big, deep breath and move one foot forward at a time? You begin by owning the truth of who you are.

You may have entrenched ideas about yourself. Some people firmly believe they truly are crazy, and they may have thought this way a long time. *What if I am certifiably crazy?* you wonder. This is highly unlikely, though we've all entertained this question at some point. *What if I compare myself to the stories in this book and still find that I'm out there?* You should expect to discover that you are different—in some ways very different. In other ways, you are much like everyone else.

Worries about these thoughts are so common that they're to be expected. We're all a little bit out there. That's the beauty of our situation. We've all got some traits that will make some uptight people scratch their heads. But you're going to learn a powerful truth—they've got their stuff too. Trust me.

So what if you discover from reading this book that you're on the edge of normalcy? That's fine. We start there. Some of your stories may be extreme. You will soon discover that we've all had extreme experiences. You'll still find freedom as you face the truth, ask tough questions, and remain open to seeing things in a new way.

"My family has been telling me for years that I'm crazy," you say. "Even asking the question about normalcy sends a shiver up my spine." Yes, and that's why I wrote this book.

"What if I read these stories and discover I'm really not like everyone else? What if my problems actually *are* bigger than others?" Yes, we've all had problems that seem bigger and worse than others' in certain areas. You'll gain a healthier perspective by reading this book. If your problems really are serious, you'll learn what others with similar problems have done to remedy them.

"What if I read the stories of others and think I've got *all* of their problems?"

This is not likely, though it is common for us to relate in some way with everyone's story. We fear our story will compare unfavorably to others'. We fear our problems really are worse than theirs, that we really do have more fears than the average person does, or that we're more difficult to get along with than normal people are. These fears are almost always exaggerated.

This book is all about gaining an accurate appraisal of our problems. It's about putting our fears and emotional issues in perspective.

Jesus proclaimed the power of letting go of our distorted view of reality and accepting the truth. "You will know the truth, and the truth will make you free," He said (John 8:32). First we come to know the truth, and then the truth sets us free.

This book is about knowing the truth—and smiling. Rather than shrink back, we're going to shout out loud. Rather than apologize, we're going to embrace acceptance. We'll hold hands, smile, laugh, and journey together on this path of discovery.

Tiptoe Through the Tulips

Are you ready to take a wild and adventuresome journey with me through the garden of our lives? Here are some of the things we'll discover as we move from feeling crazy to feeling happily peculiar:

- We all struggle with various emotional difficulties.
- Our thoughts and fears are often not as catastrophic as we think.
- Healthy comparisons keep us from feeling isolated, but faulty comparisons can kill.
- Other people are less interested in gossiping about us than we think.
- We create most of our anxiety.
- We can receive more support through transparency.
- We can almost always overcome our emotional challenges.

I hope this is good news to you. You'll be happy to see that you've created some mountains that are actually molehills. You're not on the brink of being committed, and you'll soon discover how normal you really are.

Together we'll explore how to own and embrace our challenges, smile about them, and then begin to change what we can change and accept what we cannot change. We'll talk more about this elusive condition called *normal*. We'll offer new definitions that might surprise you. Instead of accepting a definition of normal as the absence of any quirks, peculiarities, idiosyncrasies, or emotional challenges, we'll push the boundaries of this characterization. Being normal is a much broader experience than many people believe.

I'm confident that in your search for the truth, you'll discover, as I did, that you're not as crazy as you think. You'll find, as I have in my thousands of hours of professional counseling and in my personal experience in my men's group, that we all have issues.

With this understanding, you can relax. Take it easy. You have your unique story and your own history. You are where you are, and you have your own issues, and accepting this fact will make the journey much more enjoyable. Wishing you didn't have the problems you have will not help. Yes, you have issues—we all do. But together we'll discover that you're not as crazy as you've believed.

Finally, these pages will help you understand your emotional problems, accept them, and move into the healing process. You may not be as crazy as you think, but that doesn't mean you can't get better than you are. Hey, feeling good is good, but feeling better is better, right? If you discover you really do have some significant problems, you'll also find ways to put them in perspective and deal with them. No more hiding and living quietly. It's time for you to live out loud, embracing your uniqueness. This book is about acceptance, and it's also a challenge to face your problems and move into greater freedom. Let's get started!

Crazy, Normal, or Something In Between?

Sometimes you've got to let everything go—
purge yourself. If you are unhappy with anything...
whatever is bringing you down, get rid of it. Because
you'll find that when you're free, your true
creativity, your true self comes out.

TINA TURNER

I received a call yesterday from Jenny, a former client of mine whom I hadn't seen in three months. I had counseled her over several months for relationship issues. On her last visit, she was confused about whether to continue dating her boyfriend or call off the relationship. I hadn't heard from her, so I assumed she was doing fine and that she would resume counseling when she was ready.

Jenny is a vibrant, active, 35-year-old professional businesswoman and mother of three, so it was hard for me to imagine the situation she described when she called.

"I need to get back into counseling," Jenny said anxiously, her speech sounding pressured. "I don't know what happened, but I just couldn't function anymore. The stress of the business, the demands of the kids, all the pressure...I just couldn't take it."

"So what happened?"

"I dropped out. I had a nervous breakdown. I stopped running the business and let my associate take over. I just went crazy."

"What do you mean by crazy?" I asked.

"I had a nervous breakdown," she repeated insistently, assuming I'd know exactly what she meant.

Many people imagine an imaginary chasm that they must never fall into. To be standing above this ravine is to be normal, and to be down inside it is to be crazy. Many fear stepping close to the precipitous edge for fear of falling off and crashing to the bottom.

"So, tell me more about what led up to this and how you handled it."

In the few initial minutes of my conversation with Jenny, I could tell she was normal. Without a doubt, she had been through a horrendous experience, but her nerves were not broken. She was, however, obviously anxious about her experience, and she needed reassurance that everything was going to be all right.

Jenny began to tell me about the three months since her last appointment with me.

"You know I was struggling in my relationship with Terry," she said, referring to the man she had been dating. "I finally ended the relationship because he was too angry and controlling."

"Sounds like that was a good decision," I said.

"Yes, I think it was," she said sadly. "I missed him though, and the breakup was rough. Then the demands of the business got to me. I was putting in 14-hour days and then coming home to the kids, who always wanted something from me. Terry, the business, the kids...it was just too much for me to take."

"I can certainly understand that," I said. "So what did you do?"

"I asked my brother if he'd take the kids for a month, I let my associate run the business, and I tried to get rid of some of this stress. I needed to sort things out about Terry. I'd dated him for more than a year, and I thought we'd probably get married. It was a huge loss for me."

"Well, Jenny, those all sound like good decisions."

"Maybe so, but the nervous breakdown scared me," she said anxiously. "I just couldn't function anymore. I couldn't make good decisions, and I had to take some time away."

"Do you know how often people feel overwhelmed by the pressures of life and need to take time away?"

"I hope they don't feel what I felt a couple months ago."

"I bet almost everyone over 30 has experienced the feeling of having too many decisions to make and too little energy to make them. Most of us have felt that way at one time or another. Our brains feel like spaghetti and our thoughts are like molasses."

"And then they go to the hospital because of their nervous breakdown," she said emphatically.

"Sometimes they do," I replied, "but almost always they don't. What did you do after you sent your kids to your brother's house?"

"I went to the cabin. Remember me telling you about my hideaway cabin on Lake Constance? No phone and no one to bug me. It's wonderful, and I'm beginning to feel like myself again. So now I need to make an appointment and get back into counseling to sort things out. I still feel a little mixed up about Terry. And I miss my kids."

"You had a lot of stuff come at you at once, Jenny," I said. "You're a hard-working woman with a lot of pressures. But I want to reassure you that you're not as crazy as you think."

"I hope you're right," Jenny said, her voice sounding unsure. "I need to pick up the pieces of my life and move forward."

"Great," I said. "Give the office a call and get a time set up. I'll help you sort things out."

Nervous Breakdowns

What must Jenny have felt like when her life seemed to be slipping away from her? As a sharp, determined young woman, working hard to succeed at her downtown specialty boutique, she must have felt extremely anxious when she could no longer take the pressure she once thrived on.

Along with the financial pressures at work, she tried to create a healthy relationship with her boyfriend, Terry. But that didn't go well. She enjoyed her time with him, but she began to feel suffocated by his demands. In her words, she felt "trapped in a box."

Add to these pressures the stress of raising three children age six to ten. It was too much for her—probably too much for anyone.

As she felt the stress rising, she felt her grasp on her life slipping. This led to even more anxiety. Soon she was feeling anxious about feeling anxious—as many people do. She was accustomed to feeling in perfect control, so this loss of a firm grip on her life led her to become even more anxious. The result was what she called a nervous breakdown.

But Jenny wasn't as crazy as she thought. She was experiencing a crisis. Her circuits were overloaded, and she desperately needed a break. She needed to get away to clear her mind, and she was doing that quite effectively.

Many people have been right where Jenny is today. They've pushed themselves to the limit and felt as if they were losing a grip on reality. These feelings, which many of us have had at one time or another, were once referred to as a nervous breakdown. The stigma associated with this diagnosis often leaves the patient feeling even worse than before.

In the old days, medical professionals actually believed that someone who was depressed or stressed out was suffering from a disease of the peripheral nervous system. Anyone who was overloaded and couldn't think straight was given a diagnosis of melancholia, neuralgic disease, or even nervous prostration—whatever that is! The medical profession settled on the name *nervous breakdown,* which we now know is nonsense.

What was previously referred to as a nervous breakdown is in fact more likely to be a temporary phenomenon where we lose our ability to cope effectively with the stressors in our life. We find ourselves out of step with our normal functioning and experience a temporary time of emotional chaos. Frightened about this loss of functioning, we become anxious about feeling anxious, compounding the problem.

Jenny experienced a loss of normal functioning—no doubt about it. She was scared to death when she couldn't get herself to face the demands of a business she had grown from infancy several years earlier. She was frightened about her inability to meet the demands of her three children.

Jenny also struggled to understand her relationship to Terry. She wondered if she was creating their problems or if, as she suspected, he created chaos for her by his demands. These issues, combined with family and business obligations, became too much for her to manage.

What's in a Name?

The way we talk about Jenny's experience is critical. She called it a nervous breakdown, and that label made her experience even more traumatic. She felt that she had nearly lost her mind, and this was understandably terrifying.

The way you talk about your experience is also critical. Early explorers thought the world was flat, and they were concerned about sailing right off the edge into oblivion. If you picture your life the same way, you're going to be pretty frightened of any emotional chaos. If you believe you can reach a point of no return, you're going to be terrified when you feel stressed out and can't think straight. People who think this way might say they are...

losing a grip on reality

losing their minds

losing control

going nuts

going bananas

These are descriptions Jenny used to describe her situation. They are the lines I used to describe my plight many years ago when my life, as I knew it, came to a screeching halt. The parallels between Jenny's life and mine were eerie.

I too was burning the candle at both ends. I was raising a young family, working a full-time job, and studying for my doctorate. I thought I could push myself without limits. The throttle on my emotional engine was stuck wide open, and I had no brake.

I distinctly remember sitting in a crowded classroom one Saturday during a continuing education workshop. Suddenly my heart started beating faster, I began to perspire, and my thoughts started racing.

I'm going nuts, I thought to myself. *This is it. I'm going over the edge. I'm losing my grip and will be heading for a psych ward any minute.*

I frantically tried to get a grip. I tried deep breathing—without much success. I reminded myself that I was probably just feeling anxious. I told myself I could leave the room, but I was too embarrassed to slide past half a dozen people to get to the door. I looked around the room and noticed others sitting calmly, smiling, and enjoying the lecture, and that made me feel even more awkward.

All the knowledge of two graduate degrees and half of a doctorate didn't help much that day. I labeled myself in ways I encourage my clients not to. I pathologized my feelings in destructive ways.

In reality, I was experiencing anxiety—no fun, but hardly a nervous breakdown. I was experiencing the culmination of years of pushing myself too hard. My anxiety was a powerful symptom that revealed that my life was, indeed, out of control. In fact, I wasn't losing my mind. My mind is as good as ever. I did, however, lose some of my ability to tolerate enormous amounts of pressure. But that's a good loss.

We would be a lot more effective at calming ourselves if we didn't use negative, catastrophic language when we feel stressed out, but instead said things like these ourselves and maybe even to others:

> I feel overwhelmed.
>
> I feel stressed out.
>
> I can't think straight—I need a break.
>
> I'm frightened.
>
> I feel sad, discouraged, and confused.

Can you see the difference a label makes? We can talk about one experience in a lot of different ways, and the way we talk about it leads us to different reactions.

I have had years now to practice talking to myself in kinder ways. Now, when I have an episode of anxiety, I can listen to my feelings and put them in perspective. One of the primary goals of this book is to help you understand your feelings and learn that you're not as crazy as you think.

Swallowed Up

I'm working with a man who has many of the same fears and concerns Jenny has. Tad is a 40-year-old engineer at Boeing, married with two young children. Ruggedly handsome, Tad is tall with a solid build that overshadows his surprisingly quiet demeanor.

Tad handles his day-to-day functions as an engineer with aplomb. But his extended family drives him nuts. The oldest of four children, Tad has always been expected to take care of his aging parents and younger siblings who haven't been as responsible in life as he has.

Tad has felt increasingly anxious and depressed in recent months, losing sleep and feeling irritable with his wife. As we explored his feelings, he shared the following story.

"I'm not as happy as I used to be. I'm not sure what's going on, but I feel like the joy I've had all my life is slipping away. I feel like I'm getting swallowed up with darkness. Sometimes I feel like I'm losing my mind."

"Let's talk about what's happening in your life, Tad. I'm sure we can understand your symptoms in the context of your life, and together we can figure out what needs to change."

"I suppose the biggest issue is my parents," he said slowly.

"Tell me about them."

"I feel like it's always been up to me to make sure my parents are OK. They are developing more and more physical problems, and my brother and sisters don't seem to notice. My parents always call me with their problems, and it makes me furious at my siblings because they don't care. I've given up so much of my life that I don't feel like I can breathe at times. Sometimes I feel like I'm having a nervous breakdown. I wake up at night obsessing about what they'll need next. My mind is getting fried."

"Why can't your siblings help with your parents?" I asked Tad.

"Good question," he answered cynically. "They seem to think I'll always be there. I guess it's my job as the oldest kid, but it's driving me crazy."

"How do you feel about your siblings leaving everything to you?"

"How do you think I feel?" he answered, obviously angry. "It makes me mad. But any hint I give them that Mom and Dad might need some help seems to fall on deaf ears."

"Have you ever sat down and talked to your siblings?" I asked, somewhat surprised at his passivity.

"No, I haven't," he said sighing deeply. "Surely they can see that my life is getting swallowed up by our parents. You'd think they'd naturally want to pitch in and help."

"You would hope they would, Tad, but it sounds like your anxiety and feelings of craziness are a signal to you that you may need to talk not only to your siblings but possibly to your parents as well. Your role as the go-to guy needs to change."

"Yep," Tad said, appearing a bit relieved. "I think you're right. I sure can't keep going the way I have been. I'm getting resentful, and my life is suffering. I feel like I'm losing my life."

The Facts

Tad actually *is* losing his life, just as Jenny lost her life. Both allowed their lives to spin out of control, and they felt crazy as a result. But they aren't losing their minds. They aren't going crazy or losing a grip on reality. In fact, both have common symptoms of severe stress.

So the good news is that we're not as crazy as we think, but many of us still fear losing control of our minds. In fact, a 1996 study showed that about one-quarter of all Americans believed they had experienced (or had come close to experiencing) nervous breakdowns.[1] All those people believed they were on the verge of losing their minds! This number is a significant increase over results of similar studies conducted in 1957 (17 percent) and 1976 (19.6 percent).

Jenny is in good company. She, Tad, and I have all felt as if we were losing control of our minds. It is a painful (and painfully common) phenomenon.

In his book *The Anxiety Disease,* Dr. David Sheehan shares the story of an anxious young woman who was afraid she was losing her mind:

> They were sitting in the front row of the balcony in the theater. The play was boring; she noticed how quiet the audience was during one scene. Then she got a panic attack. She felt she was losing control of her mind and was going to stand up and scream in the silent theater. A moment later she thought her mind would snap: a strong impulse to throw herself over the balcony was coming over her. Since she felt she was losing control of her mind and even going insane, she feared she might act on the impulse…For weeks and months after this she felt as if she was being propelled whimsically toward a cliff and pushed close to the edge.[2]

Dr. Sheehan notes that this woman's experience of unexpected panic attacks is a typical one. He has counseled hundreds of patients who have struggled with similar experiences, though it takes some effort to reassure them that what they are experiencing is quite normal.

Myopia

A common thread runs through Jenny's story, Tad's story, and my own. We were all too isolated from others. None of us received enough helpful feedback, and all of us practiced too much critical self-reflection. Lacking healthy feedback, we are left to wonder about the way we view our lives, our families, our marriages, and our own mind. We often jump to the worst-case scenario and judge ourselves far too harshly.

In short, we lack perspective. We have no accurate point of comparison, and when we do compare ourselves to others, we often do so unfavorably.

We gain such relief when we hear someone say, "I've had that feeling too." These words can be music to our anxious ears. We're desperate to hear that we're normal after all. We feel reassurance when we realize that others have traveled the same path we have, and they have come out on a brighter side.

I commonly tell my patients that they're not as crazy as they think, and invariably when I do so, they smile and feel relief. When I offer a tidbit from my own life and struggles, they feel even greater relief.

Many of my clients express surprise and relief when I tell them I've worked a 12-step program. They assume that if I write books and speak on subjects like relationship skills and personal growth, I must have it all together.

I gently remind them that we've all got problems. We've all got families and lives and relationships that complicate matters. When we see picture-perfect people living picture-perfect lives, we must remind ourselves that this is simply an image. In fact, it is a controlled image, often intended to give a false impression. Things are never as picture-perfect as they appear.

Growing beyond our fears means growing beyond our myopia. We grow by adopting a broader point of view. In fact, the more we understand others, the more we understand ourselves. The more we learn from others, the more we can grow.

Embracing the Symptoms

Before we can change, however, we must have a clear starting point. Your starting point may be a feeling of craziness—a feeling that you somehow don't measure up, that you are odd, that you are somehow different from others.

I'll share with you what I shared with Jenny and Tad and what I've shared with hundreds of others experiencing significant stress and anxiety. They must first embrace their uncomfortable feelings— the very feelings that make them feel odd and different from others. They must look closely at these feelings and draw them close. As the saying goes, "A feeling denied is intensified." In order for a feeling to dissipate, we must first look at it closely and listen for what it might be telling us.

In just a few minutes of talking to Jenny, I heard her say something quite extraordinary. In fact, I almost couldn't believe my ears.

"I know this happened for a reason," Jenny said. "I know somehow that my world needed to collapse for me to realize what I was doing, and why I was doing it. God had to get my attention in a pretty dramatic way."

I was thrilled to hear her say that. In spite of the collapse she had experienced, and even though she'd lost an important relationship and was temporarily separated from her children, she had started to heal. She had begun to quit blaming herself and to embrace the possibilities in this crisis. She continued briefly sharing her story.

"I've felt strange and confused these past couple of months. I've lost some things that were familiar to me—it's like I'm living in a strange land. But I can see some new possibilities. I don't want to beat myself up for not seeing this crisis coming. I'm ready to let go of my old ways of doing things and start learning some new ways."

"Those are incredible insights, Jenny," I said. "You have the opportunity everyone has when they go through a crisis. You can learn from it and grow, or you can just keep doing the same things and getting the same destructive results. I know you won't let that happen."

Jenny and I talked for a few more minutes. Her voice was stronger than it had been before. I could see her resolve to find her way to a better place than where she had been.

I am impressed with Jenny. She is no different from countless others who hit brick walls and have to decide how to proceed. They can kick themselves for not having seen the wall, or they can embrace the possibilities as they lay in a heap. Certainly she is still frightened. Of course she wonders how she, a smart and determined woman, could have such a crisis. But now she'll do a better job of accepting her situation and rebuilding her life. She didn't lose her mind—only a bit of her pride, and that's not such a bad thing.

Still Not Convinced

You still may not be convinced that you're normal. That's perfectly OK. We've only begun to journey together. We've just started our group therapy.

It may help to consider where and why you have doubts. We can learn powerful lessons by embracing our doubts. See if the following statements shed some light on where you still struggle.

> My family really is crazier than anyone else's.
>
> My insecurities go deeper than other people's.
>
> I feel victimized and even persecuted by others.
>
> I'm angrier than anyone else I know.
>
> Other people say my behavior is odd.
>
> I offend others without intending to.
>
> I act impulsively, and it gets me into trouble.
>
> I can't seem to sustain a relationship.

Indeed, if you identify with any of these statements, you may have reason for concern. But that does not mean you are abnormal. Your behaviors may be on the edge of normalcy, but I can assure you that many others feel and think the same way you do.

But remember, normalcy covers a lot of ground. If your behavior or your family's behavior really is on the outer limits of normalcy, you may want to take a closer look at it. You'll have that opportunity in this book. We'll explore together some emotional problems that are normal and others that are on the outer limits of normalcy. We'll also explore the most effective ways to approach emotional problems. Labeling our issues as abnormal is rarely an effective approach to healing them. Judging them harshly and from a narrow perspective doesn't offer the gentle, loving approach needed for healing. Recognizing them and placing them in perspective opens the path to understanding ourselves so we can begin the work of healing.

The Wide Path of Normalcy

As we are beginning to discover, our primary problem is defining normalcy too narrowly. We select an image, person, or persona, decide that is normal, and try to live up to it. The problem, of course, is that our definition of normal is far too narrow.

Nearly every story of anxiety and insecurity includes a narrow definition of normal. "I should be different from who I am." "I should have handled that differently." "I can't believe I made that mistake." "Nobody else would have done what I did."

Not true. You're not as crazy as you think. Problems are normal. Facing challenges is a regular part of life. In fact, listen to what the apostle James says about difficulties:

> Consider it a sheer gift, friends, when tests and challenges come at you from all sides. You know that under pressure, your faith-life is forced into the open and shows its true colors. So don't try to get out of anything prematurely. Let it do its work so you become mature and well-developed, not deficient in any way (James 1:2-4 MSG).

Any definition of normalcy must be broad enough to include all the variations and permutations of common human behavior. We are very complex creatures, and God, in His wisdom, made us all very different. Striving obsessively to blend in, we grasp onto narrow definitions of how we are to be and behave. These narrow definitions, however, do not serve us well. We wiggle and squirm, trying to squeeze ourselves into images that don't fit us. They never will, so we end up feeling all the more insecure.

We make a mental list of qualities normal people have, and when we fall short, we feel bad. We feel inadequate and ashamed. When we struggle in marriage, we notice others who seem to never fight. When we suffer from anxiety, we fixate on people who appear to have boundless self-confidence. When we are down with the blues, everyone around us seems to bounce with enthusiastic energy. Be careful not to define yourself by these false images.

The apostle James tells us to expect problems. In fact, he shows that problems are pathways to growth. Expect to struggle, just like everyone else. We're all in this thing together.

You must fight against your tendency to compare yourself to a false image. Make every effort to broaden your definition of normal, recognizing that others are much like you. False images of normalcy are ghosts and must be treated as such. They are make-believe personas of people who don't really exist. Once we understand what normal is, we will be able to broaden our boundaries of acceptability and appreciate our unique selves. No one is perfect; no one lives without emotional struggles and difficulties. When we take a step back and look realistically at the people we call normal, we realize this. We know that many stars struggle with insecurity, lots of celebrities move from one unfulfilling relationship to the next, and plenty of powerful people succumb to addictions and suffer the consequences.

We can be thankful that Scripture offers a place for us to recover from such idolatry. In the pages of the sacred text, we see real people with real problems, and many of them discover real solutions. Their lives are not always rosy. Their families are not always relating in perfect harmony. Their lives are a bit messy, just like yours and mine.

When I feel discouraged, I remember that Elijah, the only prophet to ascend into heaven before death, also had his mood problems. When I feel anxious, alone, and strangely different from others, I remind myself of King David and his years of running from Saul. I sense his despair and grief at the loss of his son, and I cheer at his subsequent recovery.

When I feel guilty and undeserving, I remember the woman at the well, who had many failed marriages and was living with a man when Jesus welcomed her with compassion. Or the woman who was caught in adultery and brought before Jesus. The Pharisees said the law demanded she be stoned for her actions..

But Jesus bent down and started to write on the ground
with his finger. When they kept on questioning him, he

straightened up and said to them, "If any one of you is without sin, let him be the first to throw a stone at her" (John 8:6-7).

Finally, we have the character of Jesus Himself. He was perfect, but He also modeled humanity for us. This God-man exhibited an array of emotions—joy and sorrow, anger and discouragement. He dispelled any notion that we could never find acceptance. He accepts us in our fragile humanity and encourages us to grow.

Jenny has let go of a destructive relationship. She is single again and is trying to accurately define herself. Tad is learning to be something other than the dutiful son, and he's trying to relate to his parents and siblings in a more honest way. As for me—I'm still a work in progress. I'm still struggling with life balance issues as well as trying to be a more generous husband. I'll keep you posted on my progress.

We've learned about the temptation to judge ourselves harshly, inaccurately labeling ourselves. Join me as we explore the way comparisons can harm us.

Everyone Looks So Normal

*We wholly overlook the essential fact that the
achievements which society rewards are won
at the cost of diminution of personality. Many—
far too many—aspects of life which should
also have been experienced lie in the
lumber room among dusty memories.*

CARL JUNG

Last Sunday, my wife, Christie, and I went through our Sunday morning routine. Get up, shower, have breakfast, get dressed for church. As usual, I was a bit rushed as I looked into my closet, deciding what to wear. I didn't want to be too dressed up, so I put my white shirt and red and blue Jerry Garcia tie back on the hanger. Reaching for my jeans, I set them aside as well—too casual for church. Finally, after several minutes of deliberation, I settled on a pair of Dockers and a dress shirt. Not too casual and not too dressy. Still, I stopped to wonder if I should press my Dockers or if slightly wrinkled pants would be OK in church.

Out of the corner of my eye I watched Christie go through much the same routine. She first grabbed a dress but then settled on slacks and a blouse.

Arriving at our church, I noticed that nearly everyone looked as if they had conferred with one another about the dress code. Not too casual, yet not too dressy—somehow people had agreed on the appropriate attire.

33

So what was all the fuss about?

The fuss is what most people experience. We want to fit in; we want to know the rules and appear normal. Worrying about how we look and sound to others is a national pastime that robs us of much of our peace. We'll do almost anything to fit in. We may tout individuality, but most of us desperately want to blend in and then worry about how well we're doing it.

Why is blending in so critical? We want to feel normal. Normal, remember, means fitting into the norm. It's all about picturing the average person and feeling like we stack up satisfactorily next to him or her. In chapter 1, we saw that we are all pretty normal, all very much alike. Now we are going to view normal from another direction. From this perspective, we will see that when we worry about appearing normal, we squeeze ourselves into an uncomfortable mold and inhibit our growth. We might summarize chapter 1 like this: You are normal. In chapter 2, we'll see how destructive worrying about being normal can be.

As I combed my hair, Christie reminded me to hurry or we'd be late. "I hate being late," she said to me impatiently. "If we're going to be late, I'd rather not go."

"OK," I replied. "Just combing my hair, and we're out the door."

We arrived at church just a few minutes late, but we weren't so late as to be a spectacle. Others were arriving a few minutes late as well, so once again we blended in quite nicely. And that's what it's all about. Blending in. Not drawing too much attention to ourselves. Being just like everyone else.

Socialized

We make a huge assumption when we join a group of people. We assume they're largely normal, and we want to blend in or at least not stick out. As I looked around the church that Sunday, everyone appeared normal. Countless other men wore Dockers with buttoned-down sport shirts. Countless other women wore dresses or dress slacks. A few men and women wore jeans with dress shirts or blouses.

Yes, even the church has its own set of rules, which we pick up very quickly. We assume "demand characteristics" about how we are expected to behave. We understand that after entering church we are quiet. We smile at the folks sitting on either side of us, greet one another at the appointed time in the service, and leave in a dignified manner. Churchgoers in contemporary and traditional settings have their own unspoken rules.

Any group has rules like these, and they help define that group's culture. But they can also make things confusing for us in certain situations. Maybe we're new to the group and haven't learned the rules. Or maybe we expect the process to be highly personal, which often happens to be the case in contemporary churches. Or perhaps we're discovering important parts of our individuality, and we're trying to get comfortable expressing them.

That Sunday morning in church, the pastor never made an effort to connect with folks who were struggling with feelings of insecurity. He didn't mention anyone hospitalized with depression or reeling from drug addiction. He didn't comment on those who were on the verge of marital separation or divorce. He never mentioned food or gambling addictions.

No, quite the opposite. Everyone looked like everyone else, and everyone appeared to have it all together. Similar clothes and similar smiles. Everyone had taken time to conform to the image, and if that image doesn't reflect who we really are, it can throw us for a loop.

Everyone else appears to be doing fine, so I'm very reluctant to tell anyone that I'm struggling again with my work addiction. I'm not about to tell these people who have it all together that my wife and I got into a big fight on the way to church. No, this would blow my image, not to mention the unspoken rules about how to behave. Most people in our culture assume they must follow rules like these:

> Look good.
>
> Dress like others.
>
> Don't talk about your problems.

Keep your feelings to yourself.

Act like you've got it all together.

Never let them see you sweat.

Fitting In

Recently we were out of town and decided to attend a Catholic Mass. I was unfamiliar with many Catholic traditions, so I felt awkward. I was sure I stuck out from the regulars. In the foyer, people dipped their fingers into a large bowl of water and then crossed themselves. I tried this, but I don't know if I did it right. The service had some things in common with my home church, but many aspects were unfamiliar to me. Everyone seemed to know what to do but me. I started to sit when others stood; I stood when others remained seated. I quoted a version of the Lord's Prayer that was familiar to me, but it was slightly different from the one these folks used.

I felt self-conscious, wondering if people were noticing my many false moves. Could they tell I wasn't Catholic? If they could, would they welcome me anyway? What if I participated in religious rituals I didn't understand? What if I *didn't* participate in rituals I didn't understand?

Near the end of the service was the Lord's Supper—they called it the Eucharist. People filed forward, but I opted to remain seated. I wasn't sure if I should reach out for the wafer or if the priest put it in my mouth. Rather than face embarrassment, I chose to sit this one out.

These folks knew the rules of conduct—I didn't. They knew exactly how to behave, but I floundered. These folks knew how to be normal in a situation where I struggled to fit in.

Before the service was over, I began to loosen my need to fit in, and I relaxed and enjoyed the beauty of the Catholic Mass. Rather than feeling like a fish out of water, I slowly waded into the water, letting go of my self-consciousness and fears. I let go of my paranoia that everyone could see *Protestant* written all over my forehead. I let myself settle into a larger church experience, and suddenly I felt at home again and much more normal. I gave up the lines separating Protestants and Catholics, and I let myself label the larger group *Christian*.

Persona

We all want to fit in because the unpleasant alternative is to stick out. Fitting in means we're part of the norm—we're like the average Joe. We'll do just about anything to meld in with the crowd, including playing a role, or creating a false self, which has been called a *persona*. To march in lockstep to everyone else's drumbeat is to miss the opportunity to be ourselves. Our desire to look and act just like the people seated next to us may not be based on reality, but it creates enormous pressure nonetheless. We must look like them because they represent the image of normalcy, which we aspire to. Barbara Sher, author of *It's Only Too Late If You Don't Start Now*, talks about what's behind this drive to fit in:

> Approval means everything to you when you're young. If you can remember your childhood, you'll recall that approval was glorious and disapproval was agony. That makes it the most potent teaching tool for the age at which youngsters have the most to learn…This curbs your natural curiosity, which might otherwise send you off on your own explorations and put you in danger. But being restrained to this world of approval and disapproval focuses you more on rewards and punishments than on your own interests.[1]

Desperate to fit in and receive the approval of others, we develop a *persona*—a false, public self.

It's kind of crazy really, this mad push to be just like everyone else while anxiously attempting to retain our individuality. We're willing to sell our souls to appear as if we walk on water. I see you acting virtuous, so I decide I'll act virtuous as well. I see you acting most civilized, so I'll act most civilized as well. It's like a game of charades, but this is no game. It's a way to convince myself I'm not as crazy as I think. And so we broadcast messages like these:

> Of course I'm virtuous.
>
> Why yes, I follow all the rules.
>
> I would never tell a lie.
>
> I always hold my temper.
>
> I never use profanity.

It's all rather silly because we both know that we all use profanity at times. We both know that neither of us is as virtuous as either of us think. But the game provides a way for us to feel normal. Someone sets the standard, and we attempt to live up to it.

Psychologists have long studied the persona. It's an act, a public image, a false picture of who I really am, an enhanced version of the real thing. Of course the persona, or social self, has positive aspects as well. It encourages us to obey rules, to live by healthy standards, and to be loveable and likeable.

But it is too often a mask, and the mask gets heavy. Beneath the mask we know that the way we appear to others is not the way we really are. We know that instead of looking good and being good, we are only human, riddled with mistakes and idiosyncrasies. We know that beneath the facade is another person, and unfortunately, we don't let that person come out and play very often.

We can think of a few exceptions—some quite positive. To me, Brett Favre is one. I've always admired him. He loves football so much, I can understand his struggle to decide when to retire. (At the time of this writing, he's just completed his 2008 season with the Jets.)

He's always been an admitted gunslinger in football, throwing more touchdowns and interceptions than most other quarterbacks. He plays the game his way. He's not out to impress anyone. He will always be that boy from Mississippi who had a dream just like other boys have dreams. He never tries to project any other image. He can't or won't.

When Favre left the Green Bay Packers, a Reuters report described him this way: "[He is] a man who played the game like a boy. Favre's unbridled passion, boyish enthusiasm and fierce competitiveness awed teammates, opponents and fans as much as his cannon right arm."[2]

Favre did a recent ad for loose-fit Wrangler jeans, and in the ad he's seen playing a game of football with some buddies in a grassy backyard. With mussed hair and a day's growth of beard, he looks every bit like the Brett Favre we've come to admire. Loose-fit jeans. How appropriate! That's Favre—loose fit. He didn't buy into the slick persona of the well-paid, movie-star pro football player. Always the exception, he looked like a kid having fun.

Believing the Persona

We must be a bit cautious about being too critical of the persona— the civilized, socialized self who spends hours primping and preparing to blend in and look normal. After all, what's so bad about coming into church wearing neatly pressed Dockers and a buttoned-down shirt? What's so bad about following others as they anoint themselves with holy water and sit reverently in the pews, standing and sitting in respect for God, even if you have the cadence a bit off?

The trouble comes when we start confusing the persona with reality. We get into big trouble when we start thinking that others don't put their pants on the same way we do. We get confused when we convince ourselves we've got it all together or others have it all together. We forget what we learned in chapter 1—that we are all very much alike even without the persona. We lose sight of the *norm* in *normal.*

Of course, our exposure to the media doesn't help us. How in the world can we express anything but our persona when that is the only way we're taught to live? How can we think a man should be anything less than Brad Pitt or George Clooney when they are so idolized? How can a woman believe anything but her persona when she sees images of Jennifer Lopez or Angelina Jolie in perfect form day after day? These perfect people appear to live perfect lives, and the message is clear—we should be perfect too.

To Be like Mike

We cannot underestimate the power of advertising. For years I listened to commercials about Michael Jordan. He was one of the greatest athletes the world has known, and he has made much more money endorsing products and promoting his Nike line than he ever made playing basketball.

Nike spent millions betting that everyone wanted to be like Mike. Their bet paid off. Millions did want to be like Mike, wearing his jersey, his basketball pants, and of course, his Nike basketball shoes. He became something of a cult hero, and people hoped that somehow wearing his apparel would make them more like him.

Kids figured this out very quickly: *If I want to be normal, if I want to fit in, I have to buy Michael Jordan clothes.* And they were right. Buying and wearing Michael Jordan clothes did help them fit in.

Plenty of grown-up versions of the "be like Mike" advertisements tell us how to be normal. If you really want to be normal and blend in, you'll buy the latest fashions, drive the right car, wear fancy cologne or perfume, and attempt to look like the stars. But beneath the facade, you'll know you're not being true to yourself. We all know, someplace inside, that we're buying what the advertisers are selling so we can look like everyone else.

The Price of the Persona

We can usually create the right mask to look like our idols, but the mask is heavy. Ask a movie star what it is like to live with the persona of perfection day after day or even to wear a mask over her mask so she can avoid the paparazzi.

Recently Prince Harry, third in line for the throne in England, did a brief tour of duty in Afghanistan before he was pulled out because his cover was blown. Prince Harry reported that he was saddened about having to leave his buddies and the sense of normalcy he found serving his country.

One can only imagine the relief he seemed to find in relative anonymity and the regret he felt when he had to return home to be Prince Harry once again. Wearing combat fatigues, Prince Harry was able to be one of the guys. Back in London, he would once again bear the image of royalty. Living up to an image day in and day out can be exhausting.

Most of us don't struggle with the weight of stardom or royalty, but we do know the cost of trying to live up to a persona. We calculate how we should behave and then attempt to act accordingly. We determine what normal looks like and then strive for it regardless of how much the image fails to fit.

Many people try to look and act normal by wearing the cloak of conformity, but it doesn't fit them any better than a cumbersome suit of armor. Others defy it, rebelling against anything that smacks of establishment. Most of us simply strive to be like others, resenting that we have to give up so much of our true selves in the process.

Stephen is a former client. He was a 30-year-old man who acted several years younger than his age, and he'd been diagnosed with autism spectrum disorder as an adolescent. Growing up was challenging for Stephen. Fitting into an adult world has been even harder.

Thin to the point of appearing gaunt, Stephen was vaguely aware of his glaring social deficiencies. When angry with others, he pounded his fist and screamed in spite of my warnings that he could not do this in my professional office. I had to remind him, repeatedly, that he couldn't use derogatory words with me even though he was frustrated with me. He wanted to be able to say whatever he wanted whenever he wanted. Social boundaries meant little to him. He struggled to understand the specifics of these social and emotional cues.

"I want to be able to say whatever I want, Doc," he said to me repeatedly.

"I know you do, Stephen," I told him. "We all do. But that's not the way our society works. We have a certain decorum we must be sensitive to."

"Why?" he said, almost mocking me. "We all know it's not the truth."

"The truth hurts, Stephen, and I think you'd agree that we at least need to be careful of people's feelings."

"Only if they deserve it," he said boldly.

"I disagree with you," I said, beginning to see that Stephen strongly believed in the way he lived. "I think we can voice our feelings strongly, but we must always be respectful of others."

"Well, that's not the way I'm going to live," he asserted.

"Then I think you'll pay a price," I said. "I think a lot of people will be put off by you."

"Maybe so..."

Stephen lives in an unusual world. He knows he doesn't quite fit in, but he chooses not to play by all the rules. He doesn't want to bear the burden of social conformity. He knows that others are normal, but he doesn't want to pay the price to join the club.

As a result, Stephen has lived a solitary existence. Only now is he considering changing the way he interacts with others. He hopes to retain the aspects of his personality he enjoys while he finds a way to fit into society. He doesn't buy what society is selling. He wants to dress the way he likes without undue focus on fashions and trends. What you see with Stephen is what you get. No pressed Dockers with buttoned-down shirt for him. A sweatshirt, dirty jeans, and worn-out tennis shoes work very nicely, thank you.

Comparisons Kill

Stephen has some unusual opportunities. Few of us would trade our lives for Stephen's, but at least he is willing to be true to himself. Many of us would love to feel Stephen's freedom. He dances to his own drumbeat, disdaining current fashion, trends, and movements.

Because of his disorder, however, Stephen has been labeled abnormal. He is seen as peculiar, and he is aware of the public ridicule. He has grown up with cruel comments about his appearance. He is not socialized in some important ways.

Stephen's case is extreme. He doesn't function within the norm, and this is very painful for him. Slowly, however, he is coming to grips with the fact that he may always feel a bit different from others. He is slowly becoming comfortable in his own skin.

It is easy to understand why Stephen would feel abnormal. He *is* abnormal. He is abnormal because his behavior and looks don't conform to what our society has determined to be normal. He can't fit in.

What about those of us who actually fit in quite nicely but still feel as if we're on the outside looking in? We may not have a significant speech impediment or illogical thought process, but we still don't feel as if we quite fit in. What is our problem?

The answer is that we often make unfair comparisons. We put others down and find fault in them, but we also tend to believe that our problems are worse than theirs. Our marriage problems have got to be worse than others', our sex lives worse than others', our spiritual lives worse than others'…and on it goes.

Let's consider the dangers of comparing ourselves to others.

1. You will always find someone better than you. Whatever your arena of competence is, if you look hard enough, you'll always find someone better than you—and that may be painful. Comparing yourself to someone who is better than you makes you feel inferior.

2. These comparisons are often unfair. As a new piano student, I am being unfair when I compare myself to students who have been taking piano lessons for years, even if they are much younger than me. In fact, I am being unfair when I compare myself to young students even if they've been taking lessons only as long as I have because they will probably be able to pick up new habits quicker.

3. You will also find others worse than you. You might think that comparing yourself to others who cannot perform at your level would increase your self-esteem, but it doesn't always work that way. We may develop a sense of pride, but again, deep within we know that some other people are better than us. If we base our self-esteem on comparisons, we're on shaky ground.

4. When we make comparisons, we judge others. Comparisons require us to judge people rather than accept them. The Scriptures are

replete with admonitions about judging others. Judging others doesn't help us accept them and certainly doesn't help us accept ourselves. We might feel good about ourselves temporarily, but in the long run we only feel worse.

5. Comparisons push us to try to be like others. Michael Jordan can make nearly impossible moves look easy. He might inspire some people, but most people who try to learn his moves will be discouraged. Most of us are not built like Michael Jordan and will never be able to do what he does. Trying to copy him will only make us feel bad about ourselves.

6. Comparisons tempt us to copy others, so we lose our individuality. This can be used for good, as when we aspire to live up to a noble example. But more often than not, copying others pulls us away from being our true selves. Copying others means we begin acting and looking like others instead of developing our individuality.

Image Control

We know that comparisons kill, so why don't we loosen up and stop the insanity? Since when have we been so concerned with how we compare to others?

Apparently the answer to that question is since the beginning of time. David Allyn, in his book *I Can't Believe I Just Did That*, notes that we posture ourselves in much the same way that animals do. But of course, we have elevated the art.

> We rely on much more elaborate forms of image control.
> We have verbal ways of hiding our true thoughts, we have
> systems for screening our calls, we have politically savvy
> means of putting other people down.[3]

Allyn goes on to share some of the problems with image control. He says we make several mistakes that hurt us.

1. Image control stops us from taking risks, and when we don't take risks, we often assume we're in the spotlight more than we actually are.

People are not as focused on us as we think. Another way of saying this is summed up by a lesson I learned a long time ago: We wouldn't worry so much about what people think of us if we knew how seldom they do.

2. Image control often leads to drastic communication. Allyn notes that if you decide to keep to yourself, your shyness is likely to be seen as aloofness. If you decide to act tough, your act may be seen as hostility.

3. Image control robs us of opportunities to interact in ways that further our own interests. Allyn gives the example of an aspiring writer who, afraid of embarrassment, doesn't introduce himself to an editor at a party. Or a young lawyer who won't admit that he doesn't understand all the legal terms used in the staff meeting.

In my work as a forensic psychologist, I'm frequently called to be an expert witness and to defend one of my parenting or psychological evaluations. For some time I put enormous pressure on myself to have all the answers. I believed I should be able to answer any question the attorneys fired at me. The opposing attorney's job was to discredit me and my evaluation, so I often became almost ill worrying about answering every question correctly and appearing unflappable.

Struggling under this pressure, I eventually realized I didn't have to have all the answers. I learned that almost any attorney could find some fault, misspelling, or contradiction in my reports. In fact, I learned to anticipate and even predict that these sleuths would come up with some way to find fault with my report. This realization helped me see that the cost of appearing perfect was too high. The price to control another's image of me was too expensive. I was stressed out before I even took the witness stand.

Gradually I've given myself permission to use the words *I don't know.* Slowly I've learned how to admit on the witness stand that I may have made a mistake on an evaluation.

Surprisingly, giving up posturing and letting go of my need for perfection hasn't harmed my reputation in the least. Admitting inconsistencies in my findings seems only to have made me more human, approachable, and perhaps even more valuable as a professional. And admitting fallibility has certainly done wonders for my nerves!

The Problem of Pride

My problem as an expert witness had to do with my expectations for myself. This was simply another version of believing that everyone else is normal. In my case, I believed that every other expert witness was able to answer questions without anxiety or concern. I eventually realized this is not true. My colleagues helped me see the courtroom game for what it is. The opposing attorney's job is to dissect my report and find anything that can help his case.

I also made another discovery. I realized that my pride and desire for adulation are more powerful than I thought. I wanted everyone to think I gave an incredible report and performance on the stand. I wanted to impress everybody. This insight was very helpful to me, and it can be for you too. Here's how the dominoes fall.

Feeling insecure, I want admiration. I look around and erroneously surmise that other expert witnesses always keep their cool under pressure. (Wrong!) I determine to always keep my cool under pressure and compete with others to become the top expert witness. Feeling prideful, I attempt to hide my mistakes and start playing a role. I'm no longer David Hawkins, but some actor. I start to believe in this role—Dr. David Hawkins, Super Witness. In this role, I'm not allowed to make any mistakes, and I must play the role perfectly. I do reasonably well, obtain a few accolades, put more pressure on myself, and judge others who cannot do as well. I feel smaller and crazier when others do better than me. I become more detached from the real me.

J. Grant Howard, in his book *The Trauma of Transparency,* points out the root of many of our problems. He reminds us that self-centered pride was Satan's problem, it was Adam and Eve's problem, and it is our problem. "Self-centeredness is an active principle within us. Scripture refers to this inner, driving force as lust, desire, or coveting."

Howard goes on to point out that our strivings for perfection really hurt us. These strivings to be more than we are increase our feelings of craziness.

I want to be perfect. I know I am not. I've been around myself long enough to know I am weak, inadequate, inconsistent. I know painfully well that there are numerous things that bother me...I would like to live in a world that doesn't bother me. That world doesn't exist.[4]

Like Adam and Eve, I strive to be perfect. Like them, when I'm not perfect, I try to bluff my way through things, or I go into hiding. Neither are healthy responses. We all do better when we openly admit we make mistakes just like everybody else.

Sometimes we go to the opposite extreme. We practice an inverse pride when we stop thinking we're the best of the best and start thinking we're the worst of the worst. Notice the parallel between the two. In each case, we win the top prize.

I have stopped thinking I'm going to be the best expert witness on the planet. This is not to say that I don't prepare or that I don't take pleasure in a job well done. I do. But I try to keep things in perspective. I try to remember that *average* is not a bad word. (More on that later.) I remind myself that being a little above average on the bell-shaped curve of expert witnesses is not a bad place to be. Furthermore, a little failure doesn't slide me into the lowest rankings of expert witnesses.

You're not as crazy as you think. You have areas of gifting where you are above average on the bell-shaped curve. You also have areas where you're below average. On the whole, you're probably pretty doggone normal.

The Path to Perfection

We give up posturing and image control reluctantly. We all want to look good, fit in, and measure up to everyone else. Maintaining these false images helps us feel normal.

I travel frequently for my books, making radio and television appearances. I'm often asked how I apply the principles I espouse in my own family. I try to be vulnerable, sharing that in spite of all I know, teach, and write, I'm not perfect. My marriage isn't perfect. My wife and I get into petty squabbles at times. I hold grudges, even when I'm convicted not to. I can be narrow-minded and insensitive. I try to practice the principles I teach, but I realize I've not yet arrived.

I'm often surprised when I'm vulnerable. I find that the more I share my personal stories of failure, the more other people can relate to me and are willing to share their failures. Time and time again prominent Christian leaders take me aside and admit moral failures, troubled marital relationships, or failure as mothers or fathers.

At first these experiences were disturbing to me. *How could these prominent Christian leaders have such troubles? Didn't their strong Christian faith make them immune to such problems?* Of course it didn't, though many leaders seem to want to portray an image of perfection. Perhaps we parishioners even *want* them to portray this image, as unhealthy as it is for them and for us.

As I became more familiar with the inner lives of these popular Christians, I felt troubled for them. They were clunking around in heavy, ill-fitting armor, leading ministries from a perspective of perfectionism. They had to micromanage their public image, and I was one of a few people with whom they felt safe sharing the truth. Their secrets were hidden beneath their armor and were weighing them down.

And so I try to be vulnerable when I speak. I talk about my failings, old troubling habits, and immaturity. Rather than rejection and condemnation, I receive love and compassion. People can actually touch me when I take my armor off. Instead of appearing as the guy who knows it all, I'm approachable.

I share for another reason. Rather than pretending that I can become perfect, I want to become the person God made me. I grieve my failings as a father and mate because I'm a caring, compassionate, and sensitive man. When I share openly, other people feel more comfortable telling someone their secrets, and that helps them grow.

There is a better way to be accepted than trying to live up to some false image about others and ourselves. That better way is the path of transparency.

If comparisons kill, causing us to feel kind of crazy, what is our path to sanity? As others have said, the way to be perfect is to be perfectly you. This is a great moral for our lives.

Brett Favre played his own game. Stephen searches for a balance between his unbridled world of unconformity and the straitjacket world of extreme conformity. And me? I'm still looking for a way to be myself. I'm still looking for my unique voice as a writer, psychologist, son, husband, and father. Part of me still wants to fit in, and this consumes too much of my energy. Another part of me wants to take more chances, share more of my doubts and concerns, and offer my unique perspective on important matters.

In my journey, I've discovered something invaluable through my role as a psychologist and spiritual listener. I've seen powerful people humbled by incredible mistakes. I've seen humble people elevated by significant accomplishments. I've seen people with massive wealth fail to discover happiness, and others with no money find profound joy. I've worked with brilliant people who were too impressed with themselves to be a blessing to others. I've worked with people who were so consumed by their need to control that they ruined their marriages.

Appearances can be very deceiving. We dare not base our sense of normalcy or our self-esteem on what we witness on television, in the pulpit, or in the pew next to us. Our lives are far more complex, and understanding this can give us relief.

What are your secrets? What heavy armor are you carrying to hide those parts of your personality? Are you ready to exchange your armor for transparency? That is one of the most important lessons in this chapter. In the next chapter we'll learn how you can discover your true nature and live according to it.

Courageously Exploring Inner Space

What lies behind us and what lies before us are tiny matters compared to what lies within us.

RALPH WALDO EMERSON

"Space, the final frontier."

Who can hear these words without picturing William Shatner as Captain Kirk on the bridge of the Starship Enterprise? Firm and resolute, he leads his crew on their five-year mission to "explore strange new worlds, to seek out new life and new civilizations, to boldly go where no man has gone before."

We championed Kirk, Spock, Bones, and the other space travelers as they met danger head-on. Fearlessly they traveled into uncharted galaxies, challenging unknown obstacles on their quest to explore outer space. Yet Emerson's quote at the beginning of this chapter reminds us of an invaluable truth: Outer exploration pales in importance to inner space travel. Territory in distant galaxies remains uncharted, but we have uncharted territory much closer to home—within our minds.

This chapter is an invitation to journey into "inner space," where unfamiliar thoughts and feelings commingle. They seem alien because we can't name them, we don't always know where they came from, and we're not quite sure what to do with them. I invite you on a quest to understand the inner space of your thoughts and feelings—a journey no less exciting than a trip to outer space.

Who of us, in our pursuit of normalcy, hasn't been absolutely baffled when trying to understand why we do some of the things we do? Who hasn't struggled in marriage while believing that these interactions should be simple and straightforward? Who hasn't been overcome with feelings of sadness or self-doubt that seemingly arose out of nowhere? The strange aliens Kirk and friends encounter are no more baffling than the unnamed alien feelings and thoughts in our own inner space.

In outer space, even though much is unknown, we have at least a skeletal map of our solar system, our galaxy, and a few other galaxies out there. We know how to land men on the moon, study other planets, and explore at least a little bit of the universe.

With our journey to inner space—the realm of our thoughts, motives, and feelings—we are often groping in the dark. Captain Kirk expected to meet dangerous aliens, but we are often overwhelmed by our "alien" side. We don't know how to explore, label, or even talk about inner space, let alone feel comfortable there. Listen to the words of the prophet Jeremiah.

> The heart is hopelessly dark and deceitful, a puzzle that
> no one can figure out. But I, GOD, search the heart and
> examine the mind. I get to the heart of the human. I get
> to the root of things. I treat them as they really are, not as
> they pretend to be (Jeremiah 17:9 MSG).

God has evidently created our hearts and minds to be very complex, perhaps not even understandable apart from His grace. Maybe we're destined to feel a little bit crazy; maybe we'll never fully grasp how to make our minds behave. But we want to be in control, mastering inner space just as Captain Kirk took command of outer space.

You're probably reading this book because you don't like the feelings that come with an unruly mind. You've been bombarded by alien thoughts and feelings, and you want to take control. You don't want to feel crazy. Fortunately, you're an adventurer and are willing to explore inner space. But to do so effectively, you must be courageous and prepared to meet alien feelings, thoughts, and motives. You must be willing to examine parts of yourself you've abandoned long ago. These alien parts of your personality are still alive and affect the way you interact with yourself and others today.

In our inward journey, we can feel like the apostle Paul: "I do not understand what I do. For what I want to do I do not do, but what I hate I do" (Romans 7:15).

Can you relate to the apostle Paul? Do you say things that hurt others without intending to or act in ways you wished you didn't act? I certainly do.

Avoiding the Journey

Emerson and the prophet Jeremiah both had it right. The inner journey is a challenge, one we will never navigate as effortlessly as Captain Kirk seems to press his exploration of outer space. Inner space is more treacherous, and we can understand why so many avoid it. But listen to what Scott Peck says in his famous book *The Road Less Traveled:*

> A life of total dedication to the truth also means a life of willingness to be challenged. The only way that we can be certain that our map of reality is valid is to expose it to the criticism and challenge of other map-makers...[Yet] the tendency to avoid the challenge is so omnipresent in human beings that it can properly be considered a characteristic of human nature. But calling it natural does not mean it is essential or beneficial or unchangeable behavior.[1]

As I write this chapter, I've just had a fight with Christie. It was not a harsh, outward battle. It was a quiet, somber one. A stiff silence separates us.

I hate conflict. As much as I help others deal with it effectively, I still struggle with it. I don't know exactly why. Does it stem from a father whose temper frightened me? Is it a fear of my own anger? Have I not yet processed being mugged in a park by six drunken sailors when I was 19? Each feeling and memory feels both familiar and alien to me. Each seems resolved, yet jagged edges remain. This is the way it is with most of us—past memories, events, and traumas all impact the way we react today.

Our fight began early this morning, and it is now midafternoon. Christie asked a favor of me, and I declined. My tone was sharp, and she reacted in kind. My defensiveness triggered her defensiveness. Like sparks in dried grass, our words quickly ignited our tempers. We called a time-out, but we haven't spoken for several hours.

A thousand things run through my mind. I begin by justifying my actions, of course. Then I try to understand what I said and how I said it. Then I justify my actions—again!—and wonder why she has to be so sensitive. And then I recognize I am also very sensitive, and that is one of the things we admire about each other.

I've spent the day at a café writing. As Peck says, we find ways of avoiding the truth. I don't want to escalate matters, and I want to be in my best frame of mind when I call her. I want my heart to be at peace and ready to reconcile, but I don't want to face any harsh realities.

It's all a bit of a muddled mess. This is what we were taught in Psychology 101—the classic approach-avoidance conflict. I want to come close, but I push away at the same time. I want peace and I want to blame—simultaneously. These jangled thoughts and feelings make me feel crazy. How can I possibly understand my deepest motives? How can I understand her motives?

I take some comfort in reminding myself that my thoughts and feelings are normal. I may *feel* crazy and a bit out of control, but this messiness is the stuff of relationships. I know this from working with people every day. I see their distress and frayed nerves, their distorted thoughts and self-destructive actions. I walk with them through this alien territory.

At moments like these we do well to shift back to what we know for sure. Here is a short list for me:

- I love my wife.
- Being in relationship is better than winning an argument.

- A heart of reconciliation is better than rigid legalism.
- I am not perfect.
- I want reconciliation.
- I know how to seek reconciliation, and I can be caring, forgiving, loving, and kind.
- I can also be small, demanding, perfectionistic, and distant.
- I want the former, not the latter.

Embarking on the inner journey requires courage. When I make the call to Christie, I must be prepared to be challenged. I may feel embarrassed, frustrated, and even angry again. I must be prepared for seemingly alien feelings to arise in me, and I must face them courageously. I may discover aspects of myself I'd rather not know. This is only one of the challenges of exploring inner space.

Ignoring Your Feelings

We've all been taught to ignore our feelings. Contemplation is not encouraged in Western culture, so many of us are ineffective when exploring inner space. Some people suggest exploring inner space is for sissies or a waste of time. They say, "Ignore your feelings, and they'll go away," and in one way they're right. Ignore your feelings, and eventually you will not recognize them or know how to talk about them. But your feelings *will not* go away.

Ignored feelings, thoughts, and memories lay submerged in a sea of subconsciousness, waiting to erupt at unlikely times. Like a balloon held under water, these restricted feelings shoot to the surface when released by some external event. These seemingly alien feelings and thoughts continue to exist when we ignore them. In fact, they become intensified over time, and that adds to our feelings of craziness.

I've had a longstanding friendly discussion with my sons over emotional matters. Both are trained in the hard sciences as physicians.

Their schooling emphasized physical maladies, not emotional and spiritual issues.

But their training, in spite of the heavy emphasis on anatomy, physiology, and disease processes, would be incomplete without understanding the human element—aspects of dis-ease that cannot so easily be seen. Broken bones can be X-rayed and reset. Cancerous tissue can be radiated or removed. But what about the ache of loneliness or the broken heart and the impact they have on well-being?

Both Joshua and Tyson have been forced to pay closer attention to the role of emotions and to examine the mind-body connection. Issues of the soul and spirit are woven into our physical being. These places of inner space are not easily seen or diagnosed. To explore these areas requires a keen sense of presence, time, and understanding.

My sons are learning that bedside manner and an attentive ear are sometimes the most potent remedies they can offer. They understand that people's mind-set toward their illness is as critical to their healing as are their X-rays and blood tests. Joshua and Tyson have learned the mind has the power to make the body sick, and it has the power to heal.

Unfortunately, some Christians teach people to treat emotions as aliens and to reject them when they are unpleasant. My Sunday school teachers used to show my friends and me a picture of a train, suggesting that faith was the locomotive driving the train, facts comprised the body of the train, and feelings brought up the rear in the caboose. We were taught that we could count on our faith, but our feelings were fickle, and we should regard them with suspicion or even dismiss them.

Exploring inner space and the world of our feelings is not a ride in the caboose. In fact, our feelings can be an incredibly powerful source of information and even a way for God to talk to us. When our worlds are particularly confusing, our feelings can help us see what is important to us and why we do some of the things we do.

Consider how the biblical narrative would read if we anesthetized the emotional life of the characters. Moses would never have broken the first stone tablets when he saw Israel's idolatry. David's psalms would be flat. He would never be frightened, angry, or mournful, even in the face of Saul's death threats. And he certainly wouldn't dance for joy before the Ark. Ruth's story would be boring. Living as a widow in a foreign land would be no big deal. Elijah would never have fled in fear of vengeful Jezebel or heard God's still, small voice at the mouth of a cave. Esther wouldn't have felt a thing when she risked her life to save her people. Jesus would never have wept at the loss of his friend Lazurus, had compassion on the sheep without a shepherd, or been "full of joy through the Holy Spirit" (Luke 10:21). And He wouldn't have sweat blood in Gethsemane.

No, to understand Scripture and the stories of the biblical characters, we must pay close attention to their feelings. We must feel what they feel—their fear and courage, their anger and compassion, their sorrow and joy. Then we can appreciate that Jesus came alongside His friends in their celebrations and in their mourning.

Whenever people are critical of their own emotional life and seem to believe that they should somehow rise above their emotional experience, I take them to Scripture. There I find someone who has walked where they have walked, hurt in a way that they have hurt, and overcome obstacles that they can overcome.

Permission

One of the primary reasons we don't explore inner space is that we haven't given ourselves permission to take the journey. We tell ourselves to stay away from unfamiliar thoughts, feelings, motives, or actions. Except for the few who willingly explore dreams—distorted aspects of daily life—we refuse to risk meeting the resident aliens in our minds. We deny ourselves the opportunity to learn more about who we are. Before you can embark on the journey to inner space, you'll need to give yourself permission to enter this somewhat forbidden territory. I invite you to learn more about yourself than you've ever known.

What if we took a deep breath and sat quietly, journal in hand, and began taking note of our thoughts and feelings? What if, instead of being afraid of what we might find there, we had an explorer's mind—one of inquisitiveness?

"Hmm. That's a peculiar thought!" we might note.

"Wow! I wonder why that memory of my grandfather is coming back to me right now."

"Why does this movie make me feel so sad?"

When we give ourselves permission to meet these unconsidered feelings and thoughts, they're no longer so alien. Let me offer an example.

Just last night Christie and I were having dinner out. She began talking about our children and some of their difficulties. On one level I simply listened and enjoyed the meal. On another level I noticed my mood darken. I felt a sense of sadness come over me. For a moment I tried to push the feeling away, but then I decided to simply say what I felt.

"I'm sad for Justin, Rita, Kira, Dee, and Colin. I'm concerned about Josh and Jacqueline, Tyson and Jordana, too. I feel sad for them, and for you."

Christie's eyes welled with tears, and immediately I began crying as well. Slightly aware that we were in a public restaurant, I decided it was more important to attend to our feelings than stuff them away or offer inane platitudes.

After dinner, we walked back to our hotel quietly, still feeling sad in spite of a fabulous meal out. Christie and I stopped again, held hands, and prayed for each of our children. We felt better.

We could have stuffed our feelings or talked ourselves out of our sadness. We could have given our feelings a few moments and then rushed ahead into a lighter topic. We didn't. We gave ourselves permission to experience our feelings and thoughts and to attend to them.

Emoting Is Not Selfish

For others, the notion of exploring and sharing thoughts and feelings feels embarrassingly self-centered. Painstakingly writing out our daily thoughts and feelings and possibly even our nighttime images is too tedious. We question the value of sharing our feelings with others. We hope to leave our feelings in the alien world of our unconscious, mistakenly believing they'll stay there and leave us alone. Cheryl Richardson makes this note in her book *Take Time for Your Life:*

> Making your self-care a priority can be scary, even offensive, at first. Yet, as you begin to filter your decisions through the lens of extreme self-care, you'll find that your nagging inner voice becomes a strong ally in helping you make better choices.[2]

One reason we feel abnormal is that we listen to other voices instead of our own. When we listen to a cacophony of voices, we can easily feel lost in a crowd. People are all around, and we need not become reclusive to pay attention to our inner space. But the din of other voices will obstruct the clarity of our one clear voice unless we focus our attention.

Listening to your self requires a singular purpose. It requires focus as well as loving, careful attention to your self. This is not as easy as it sounds. Richardson offers a warning:

> Initially, you may feel some resistance to being selfish. You might feel guilty, uncomfortable, uncaring, unspiritual, or concerned about the reaction of others. But tell your friends and family that you've decided to take care of your "Self." They may very well react (as a matter of fact, you can expect that some of the people in your life will give you a hard time), but remember, your life is at stake.[3]

What is your initial reaction to the notion of giving yourself permission to listen to your self? Does it sound a bit New Agey? Perhaps it conjures up the notion of contemplating your navel. It is actually anything but that. Listening to your self is simply making friends with your self, probably after years of feeling estranged and alienated from your thoughts and feelings. In a world that celebrates being available to others, giving yourself permission to be true to your self is unique.

The poet E.E. Cummings once said, "To be nobody but yourself, in a world which is doing its best night and day to make you everybody else, means to fight the hardest battle which any human being can fight; and never stop fighting."

The Perilous Journey

Another reason many don't take the inner journey is that it can be perilous. Who really wants to know their dark and secretive motives? Who wants to face the alien and sometimes aggressive thoughts and feelings they have pushed aside? What if we learn things about ourselves we'd rather not know? Maybe we'll only increase our fears that we're not so normal after all!

Cummings had it right. The battle to be uniquely yourself may be the hardest battle you'll ever fight. Your world, including your family, your mate, and even your friends, will try to make you into what they want you to be. You must resist. You will have to counteract the tremendous pull to be like everyone else, to bleach out troubled feelings, and to anesthetize your pain.

Cassandra wrote to me not long ago. She was venomously angry but not with her mate, her friends, or herself. She was furious with her church, and this frightened her. Cassandra's husband is the church's pastor. Here's her story.

"I cannot be myself in my church. Everyone expects me to be a certain way. There is a model for being a pastor's wife. I am supposed to dress a certain way, act a certain way, and always be available to anyone who needs me. I've done that in the past, and I just about died. Now I am just trying to be me. I have a life outside church, and the people in the church don't like it. They disapprove of me, and of course, that upsets me. I want to be liked, and I want my husband to be successful. It's like he will be successful only if I give in to their desires. I better sing in the choir, teach a Sunday school class, and develop the women's ministry. But that's not me. What can I do?"

Cassandra had a real fight on her hands. To be successful as the wife of the pastor, she was expected to be a certain way. She had to make some difficult decisions. Should she sing in the choir even though this was not her gift? Should she head up the women's ministry program even though this did not fit her and she had no passion for it? Or should she pursue her calling as a graphic designer?

Cassandra battled within herself. One voice cried for her to join the crowd and be what the church wanted her to be. *Find friends in the church, meet the needs of the church, and help your husband be successful.* This sounded like the "Christian" thing to do.

Another voice resisted, creating tension within. *No, you're meant to be an artist. God gave you a gift and a passion for creativity. You speak through forms, images, and colors, not words.*

For years, Cassandra pushed these alien feelings away, but now she couldn't silence them any longer. With growing resentment, she felt she could no longer tolerate the clamoring voices of others telling her what to do. She was experiencing a true identity crisis.

Mary Oliver is an acclaimed poet who has touched many lives. Any discussion of exploring inner space would be incomplete without mentioning her poem *The Journey,* in which she eloquently shares how the world will desperately try to mold us into its image. People want us to conform to their expectations. Sometimes these expectations are obvious and annoying; other times they are more subtle, yet we feel their tug. Conform. Fit in. Be what others want you to be. But Oliver shares the power and majesty of standing firm, grasping fervently to your one and only life. It is yours to manage. Your individuality is one of the only things you possess. For all of your quirks and idiosyncrasies, you are you and must hold onto your self tightly.

Oliver says the only life we can save is our own. This initially sounds as if it goes against traditional Christian beliefs that say we must lose our life in service to others. In fact, Scripture says that in order to find our lives we must lose it. Are these two messages mutually exclusive, or do they actually work together?

Cassandra found out the hard way that the way she was losing her life in service to others meant only one thing: losing her life and feeling crazy. Fortunately, her inner journey led her back to herself and to her gifts. She discovered that when she attended to and embraced her true gifts as a designer, she was able to use her gifts with others. Her joy returned. She discovered the only way to feel normal was, as Scott Peck advised, to be rigorously honest with herself. She found she could effectively serve others only from within her calling—not from what others wanted her to be.

Embracing Your Self

This business of celebrating your self is news for many. Many people live their lives assuming they have already established their self, so they think the inner journey is unnecessary. The idea of taking an inner journey, of exploring thoughts and feelings, is foreign to them.

But most people have never attempted an in-depth inner journey, and as a result, lots of people have no idea who they really are. They lack a cohesive sense of identity primarily because they've never taken the time to fully understand and embrace who they are.

You may feel crazy because you've tried to be too many things to too many people. You've assumed everyone else knew what was best for you—what you should think, feel, want, and do—and so you let others direct your life. It may be time for a change!

Several years ago I decided I wanted an Irish setter. I love their rich, red coats, their regal heads held high, and their stately, long legs.

Without research, I purchased a pup with long, gangly legs and feet nearly the size of its head. He was absolutely adorable, and it was love at first sight.

After bringing the puppy home, I enjoyed the first few hours of playing with him, allowing him to get to know our home.

And then it began. This pup began acting like an Irish setter. He began bouncing all over the place in spite of my protests that it was now time to sit still. It was time to stop chewing on table legs and other pieces of furniture and act like a well-disciplined animal.

The next several weeks were challenging to say the least. I had expected a delightful, loving dog that would lie at my feet all the time. I wasn't prepared for a dog that wanted to run and run and run. I could feel the tension in his body when restrained—he was built to run.

I wonder if there are similarities between tuning into a dog and being sensitive to a person. Before choosing a dog, the smart owner does some research. She compares a dog's temperament with her own to see if they are suited for one another. When I tried to make a cocker spaniel out of an Irish setter, I was in for trouble. Similarly, when I expect myself to act outside of my temperament, I should expect to be frustrated.

As a psychologist, I'm interested in why we do what we do. How can there be so many variations of this one human species?

Our son Justin is a case in point. According to the Meyers-Briggs Type Indicator, a temperament analysis, Justin would be an Introvert/Intuitive/Feeler/Perceptive. In layman's terms, he's one unique breed of cat.

Justin is a delightful young man. He is a sensitive, thoughtful musician. He loves obscure movies and books. He dresses from thrift stores with sweater vests, faded jeans, and motley hair. He is perfectly comfortable in his own skin.

If you tell Justin he should shop at Nordstrom, he'll think you're nuts. If you tell him to trade in his old, dented Suzuki for a new car, he'll ask you why. If you try to make him something he's not, he'll resist you.

If, however, you decide to learn from him, you'll become enriched in the process. You'll discover that he has embraced his very unique individuality. He's not trying to be an Irish setter. He's a loveable cocker spaniel and will shower you with love all day long. When he starts talking about some obscure band, book, or movie, you quickly learn what excites him.

After months of failure and frustration, I learned that I had to give my setter room to run. I had to be sensitive to his energy and needs. I had to let him expend his energy and be true to his innate temperament, and after he finished, he could enjoy lazing around some.

You are on a unique journey, one that no one can take for you.

Your journey is the discovery that you are unique and that you interact with your world in very unique ways. Efforts to make others see things your way are bound to be met with resistance, and trying to be what others want you to be is a sure road to feeling crazy. We're all unique and need to become comfortable in our own skin.

Embracing Imperfections

When we courageously explore inner space, we inevitably find surprises in our closets. We've erringly labeled these alienated aspects of ourselves *skeletons,* but in fact they are simply parts of ourselves we've pushed away. They desperately need love.

Who can dare open the door to the inner closet without finding a thief, a liar, a braggart, or all three? Who won't find a coward and an insecure weakling? Who won't find a villain and a victim wrapped in one? These aspects of our personality may be disdainful, but they need loving attention.

When you begin your inner journey, be prepared to find all kinds of personalities made into a most beautiful mosaic of imperfections. You will find yourself beautiful only if you approach this journey knowing full well that you are a million personalities all made into one. To believe anything different is foolish.

One of the therapies I enjoy most is the exploration of our different, imperfect parts. In fact, it's called *parts therapy.* In this kind of therapy, we expect to find many different imperfect selves. Where we find a hero, a fearful one is right behind. Where a courageous one appears, a coward also steps out.

When we explore our selves, we are deluded if we believe that we must be only one part. We will be very disappointed if we think we should have one clear thought, one singular emotion, with no confusing loose ends. Uncomfortable with these fragmented feelings, we push away aspects of our selves, leading to alienation and a feeling of craziness. We falsely believe that we must fit together perfectly with no jagged edges.

During my own personal therapy and group therapy, I learned about my different inner parts. I learned that I felt neglected by my parents as a youngster, as both worked demanding jobs. Even now those old feelings of rejection can be triggered.

I also learned that I too can be rejecting. As much as I hate being rejected, when I'm angry I can push people away—a trait that is self-destructive. Wanting comfort and care, I may push Christie away if I feel neglected. You can see how my different parts act in different ways, leading to confusion at times.

Most important, I learned that I'm a work in progress. I don't understand all my feelings, all my thoughts, or all my actions. I'm learning to give myself permission to be imperfect. Joy Browne writes about this kind of experience in her book *The Nine Fantasies That Will Ruin Your Life:*

> The need to be perfect is a terrible burden. It means there is no rest, no serenity, only striving and failing, since perfection can't change and to be alive means to change. So, even if it were possible to be momentarily perfect, that would be the end of the line—as a verb, "to perfect" means "to finish." The gnawing sense of imperfection can taint the simplest pleasure and the greatest triumph.[4]

Most of us intellectually agree that perfectionism can be harmful, but still we strive for perfection in most of what we do. As a result, we're forever haunted by the possibility of being exposed. What if my friends or colleagues or fellow churchgoers discover that I…

am a fraud

have a bad temper

sometimes cheat

sometimes lie

have a criminal record

have been sexually abused…

We carry around fears of exposure like so many rocks in a backpack. We applaud vulnerability but don't practice it. We champion acceptance but don't really give people a chance to experience it. We boldly assert forgiveness but don't get close enough to others to give or receive it.

To embrace your temperament is one thing, but to embrace unpleasant qualities in your personality is something quite different. What are you going to do with those qualities that are not so admirable? Embracing your self includes coming to grips with a lot of imperfections. This is much easier said than done.

Beauty in Brokenness

Christie finds pieces of sea glass in the gravel and sand near our home. She walks slowly and cautiously along our beach in search of these relics. The glass that someone threw overboard as refuse becomes her treasure. She carries these colored bits of glass home, puts them in a vase, and places the vase on a windowsill. The pieces fall into place, and the different shapes, hues, and sizes create a mosaic and beautifully reflect and refract the sunlight. Sometimes she places fresh flowers in these vases, and sometimes she simply leaves the assortment of glass alone.

Our lives are like those beautiful broken pieces of glass. Time has ground down some of our edges and made them smooth. Other shards still have sharp edges that cause us pain. In time, and with proper reflection, they too can become sanded and smooth. Our brokenness, accepted and even loved, can be part of a fabulous, colorful mosaic. But this requires loving *all* the pieces of our selves—even the ones we'd rather not own.

I've come to believe we can only courageously explore inner space if we do so with a soft eye. If we are too critical of ourselves, as others have been with us in the past, we won't risk being vulnerable. If we judge ourselves too harshly, as others have judged us in the past, we won't open up, even to ourselves.

What if you could be assured you were a beautiful mosaic? What if you could be assured that the mixture of broken pieces of different hues, sizes, and shapes could make a wonderful work of art? Would you then love your self and feel a little less crazy? I think so.

Soulful Listening

Discovering who you are is easier said than done. Many voices are telling you where to live, what activities to pursue, and how you should be. Very few voices are applauding you for following your dreams or listening to the small, inner voice that is part of your fragile self.

I want to invite you to use a powerful tool in the inner journey. I call it *soulful listening*. This is the delicate practice of listening to your heart. It means getting real with your self regardless of how painful or life-changing the experience may be. Imagine listening to your self for these themes:

- What is trying to give birth in me today?

- What is dying?

- What changes are being demanded of me at this time in my life?

- What do I hear God calling forth in me?

Soulful listening means listening to the voice of your soul—often an alienated part of your self. This means listening for more than simply the facts of your life.

One middle-aged woman recently told me that she was considering going back to college and that her husband wasn't happy about it. I could hear both excitement and fear in her voice. Telling me the facts of the matter hardly spoke the depth of her desire to finish her degree or the angst she felt about upsetting her husband.

As we spoke more about her wishes, she told me she had always wanted to teach, and she had recently heard that schools were looking for teachers and teaching assistants. Now that their children were grown and she had more time, she felt this goal was within her reach. Her husband, however, seeing retirement in the next ten years, didn't like the idea and resisted her wishes. She was in a quandary as to how to proceed. She wanted to be true to her desires but didn't want to jeopardize their marriage. They would need to have much more conversation and negotiation about how their desires can intersect, each listening soulfully to the other.

Soulful listening involves paying special attention to the subtle nuances of your life. It means listening to the ongoing story of your life and noticing how it is changing over time. Gail Saltz, in her book *Becoming Real,* explains that this is part of the process of becoming real.

> Becoming real happens when our stories start to collapse. When our orderly worlds become erratic. When we begin to see patterns of behavior we don't want in our lives, we are forced to see beyond the fiction...becoming real happens when we accept ourselves in our totality—the good, the bad and the ugly, the strengths and weaknesses.[5]

Lewis Carroll's *Alice's Adventures in Wonderland* is a humorous story of a girl in search of herself. Her story is our story.

> "Who are *you?*" said the Caterpillar.
> This was not an encouraging opening for a conversation. Alice replied, rather shyly, "I—I hardly know, sir, just at present—at least I know who I WAS when I got up this morning, but I think I must have been changed several times since then."

This process of introspection, of seeing the truth of the matter, requires courage. If we look closely, we'll see that we are in the process of change. We must be willing to see things we'd rather not see, feel things we'd rather not feel, and make changes we'd rather not make. But being real is a sure path to feeling a lot less crazy.

Journaling

Another invaluable habit to cultivate on your courageous journey is journaling. Putting into words what you feel, what you think, and what you want, on a daily basis, allows you to observe the fluctuations in your life. Journaling invites you to meet and befriend parts of your self that you've alienated.

I consider journaling a way to carry on an ongoing dialogue with myself. It's as if I awaken every day and ask, *David, how are you today? I'd like to hear. What you feel, think, and want are important to me. Please tell me.*

I proceed to answer as if my journal has caring, listening ears for what is happening within me. Anything of importance is likely to become an ongoing theme in my life. If something is important, and many things are, I will begin thinking about them, dreaming about them, and even daydreaming about them.

As I've already shared, observing my feelings about something helps me understand what is important to me. If I consistently feel sad about something, for example, I probably need to grieve some loss taking place in my life. If I consistently feel angry, perhaps I'm allowing some important boundary to be repeatedly violated. I wouldn't know about these critical needs if I didn't journal or somehow take notice of the stirrings inside me.

I also use my journal to encourage a helpful dialogue between the parts of myself. For example, I might want to participate in some activity, but I might also feel reluctant and want to take a break from it. Writing out both sides of the emotional equation, or even writing out a dialogue between these two different parts, helps me make a decision about the matter.

Talking It Out

Journaling doesn't work for everyone. Some desperately need to share their heart with a real-life person. They need an available friend who cares what they're thinking and who will journey through the morass of troubled feelings, the muck of thoughts not well assembled, and the feelings in disarray. They need someone who will simply hold their hand as they sort through their scattered collection of broken glass.

Some people want a professional to serve in this role. A friend is helpful, but a professional has heard it all before and can provide objectivity. A professional can offer those comforting words, "Others feel that way too."

Many people also find a comforting home in prayer. Sitting alone in your special prayer room, a hallowed sanctuary, or in your quiet time with the Lord, you echo the words of the psalmist: "O Lord, my Rock and my Redeemer."

We've seen the importance of taking the journey to inner space and learned that this is critical to discovering how normal we really are. In our next chapter, we'll see that our feelings of abnormality can actually be helpful for us.

4

You Really Want
to Be Normal?

*The miracle is not to fly in the air or walk on the water,
but to walk on the earth.*

Chinese Proverb

By now you're beginning to understand that this thing called *normalcy* is a bit elusive. We're forever searching for normal, wanting to be part of it, comparing ourselves to it, and yet we feel as if we fall short of it. The very process of striving to be normal makes us crazy!

You're also beginning to understand that unhelpful comparisons can kill. We grab hold of an image or seize a set of expectations, and then we measure ourselves by those expectations. The very act of trying to be what others expect us to be, however, also makes us dizzy. We quickly lose sight of the unique individual God created each of us to be.

You've begun the process of courageously exploring inner space—recapturing alienated parts of yourself. You're bravely looking in old closets for your skeletons, and you're loving them back into your self. In your search, you're seeing your faults and peculiarities with new objectivity.

Even though you have come such a long way, you may continue to doubt that you're really normal. Your problems remain magnified in your mind. Your unusual traits still loom large. That's actually good because we need to take a turn in the road.

We've been assuming that we all want to be normal, as if that is

71

our barometer for well-being. We want to fit in because we think that will make us happy. But perhaps we've been moving ahead too quickly. Let's slow down and rethink a few things.

During your inner journey, you undoubtedly have discovered aspects of yourself that you like and other parts of yourself that you wish would just go away. Perhaps you're still tempted to get out a huge bucket of Clorox and bleach the stains out of your history. A bright and shiny white personality may still look pretty good to you.

But that's not the way things are in the real world. It never has been and never will be. We're all speckled. We're all spectrums of light and dark and every hue in between. I hope the analogy of your personality as a beautiful mosaic has helped you to appreciate and love these mottled and possibly discarded parts of your personality.

As a kid, I was obsessed with fitting in. I hated the fact that I had "alligator skin," or what I later discovered was eczema. I disliked the fact that I couldn't breathe like others, discovering later that I also had asthma. I hated that I didn't excel in any sport—I was always average.

I loved the fact that I could spell better than other students and that I seemed to have a knack for writing. I enjoyed my outgoing personality. I clung to these traits and tried to push other traits out of my awareness. For all the pros and cons, I wanted to be just like everyone else. I would gladly have given up my trumpet playing prowess to dribble the basketball as well as some other kids. I would quickly have traded my blond hair for straight teeth and clear skin. I so badly wanted to trade unpleasant traits for lovelier ones.

I meandered through primary and secondary school without too many scars, always obsessing about just being average. This belief began to crumble when I went to college and studied the bell-shaped curve, in which the vast majority of people fall into the middle of the pack.

You might recall that when we compare our grades, income, eye color, height, weight, hair color, and just about any other measurable trait of personality, practically all of us fall within the mean. Statistically, nearly all of us are average.

All of a sudden, sitting in my statistics class on the campus of Western Washington University in 1974, I realized that *normal* and *average* have nearly the same meaning. Looking around, I began to size up the class. Nearly 70 percent of us would obtain Cs. Seventy percent of us were white Anglo-Saxon Protestants. Seventy percent of us came from families making essentially the same income, lived in the same kinds of houses in the same kinds of neighborhoods, and had parents who worked in the same kinds of jobs. We took the same kinds of vacations, had the same kinds of friends, played the same kinds of sports, spoke the same language, and had the same extracurricular interests. You get the statistical point.

To be normal means, in large part, to be average. You fit in nicely, blending in with others. You think like them, dress like them, and even start to feel the same feelings they do. In fact, pretty soon you may even wonder if you are distinct from them in any way whatsoever.

And you're sure you want to be normal?

Picasso

My wife and I recently celebrated our wedding anniversary in Barcelona, Spain. Barcelona, as you may know, was the place Pablo Picasso spent many of his formative years and officially declared himself a painter. Everywhere we went, we saw posters of the city's famous son. But Picasso wasn't always celebrated and beloved.

Pablo Ruiz was the son of Jose Ruiz, an art teacher and painter, and Maria Picasso Ruiz. Picasso showed his talent for art at a very young age, during his "blue period," while living a Bohemian lifestyle. He learned everything he could from his father but then abandoned those techniques, branching out on his own.

Picasso refused to follow the mainstream in art. He couldn't be average or normal. He felt compelled to follow his heart, which led him to strange and unusual places. Picasso explored new directions in art, grew his hair long, wore strange clothes, and incurred the wrath of his father, who believed Pablo was wasting his talent.

Feeling too constrained in his home town of Málaga and his newly adopted city of Barcelona, Picasso moved to a new city and country, where his soul longed to be—Paris, which at that time was the center of the art world. He lived in a cold, run-down building, painting constantly, sometimes surviving for days on only a piece of bread.

Picasso made some difficult decisions. Instead of following his teachers, he explored work in sculpture, graphic arts, ceramics, mosaics, and stage design. He pioneered work in cubism, and eventually his works were celebrated in museums and private collections around the world.

Imagine this vagabond roaming the streets of Paris and eking out a living as a starving artist. Imagine the voices in his head: *Get a real job!* Can you hear it? Can you empathize with the pressure he must have felt?

Picasso became famous because he rejected the formal rules of art. He mastered realistic painting at a young age and then experimented with other ways of seeing the world and expressing what he saw. He invented new styles and worked with new material. He even worked with junk, creating a bull's head out of parts from an old bicycle.

Picasso clearly danced to a different drummer. He rejected an opportunity to be normal and chose to become an eccentric painter. Rather than follow in others' footsteps, he chose his own path. We can be thankful that Picasso followed his passion, as did Gaudí, Degas, da Vinci, and hundreds of other rebels. Where would we be without these individuals, who colored outside the lines of conformity?

Outside the Lines

When most of us were in elementary school, we were under incredible pressure to conform. We were not asked to express what was inside. Somehow those urges were deemed abnormal. Normal was what everyone else was doing. Normal was a prescribed way of doing things—what the teacher had been trained to extract from us. We were taught to color inside the lines.

Picasso and other geniuses gave themselves permission to express their passions. Were they more creative than you and me? Perhaps yes and perhaps no. Might they have simply allowed themselves permission to color outside the lines?

In *Fingerpainting the Moon: Writing and Creativity as a Path to Freedom,* Peter Levitt shares the story of standing alone in a public garden. After a brief time a friend came up to him and said, "You know, there's room for us."

Levitt writes, "As she spoke she swept her hand in a gentle arc to include all the various forms of life before us…'If there wasn't room,' she said in a conspiratorial smile, 'we couldn't be here at all.' And then she really smiled."

This message touched Levitt deeply. "As I watched her walk away, I felt the true gift she had given with the depth that took me by surprise."

Levitt believes we all have an endless bounty of creativity within, the flow of which is too often cut off by never-ending obstructions. When we strive to be normal, we disrupt our natural creativity and imagination. Levitt suggests we follow a different course.

> Our imaginations freely give us what they want us to have
> at any given moment for reasons of their own. This is the
> source of permission that cannot be denied. Our task, then,
> is to recognize and accept this permission—and the freedom
> it implies—as part of our life force, and to find a way to
> use these gifts to further express our lives.[1]

The life force Levitt refers to, in my opinion, is the Spirit of God moving inside us. God has created each of us to be creative. In fact, Genesis 1 may indicate that God designed us to be cocreators with Him. But accepting this invitation will take courage and will mean coloring outside the lines—well beyond the expectations and limitations that other people would have us accept.

Lockstep Living

They fill my office. Middle-aged men and women who are tired of their lives. They have become what society has labeled normal. They have a house in the suburbs, 2.3 children, two incomes, two weeks of vacation, two cars, and too much boredom. It has all become too much. Perhaps too much normalcy.

Hal was such a man. A robust, rugged 52-year-old with a wispy silver beard, he had achieved everything he had set his sights on 30 years earlier. Happily married with two grown children, he was surprised by his growing depression.

Hal came to see me very reluctantly. As a doctor, he prided himself in understanding both the inner and outer workings of a person.

"I don't know what's the matter," he said firmly to me at his first visit. "Everything in my life is fine. I'm happily married, and our kids are attending college. We have more time and money than I could have hoped for. We attend a nice church, have some nice friends, and live in a nice home."

"Sounds very nice," I said, echoing his flat tone.

"Yep," he said, ignoring my humor. "It is very nice, so I'm not sure what's wrong with me. I don't know why I'm not happy. I have what everyone else wants."

"Tell me more about how you're feeling, Hal."

"I feel depressed," he said slowly. "At least I think it's depression. I don't sleep like I used to. My appetite is affected, and so is my sex life. And my practice is starting to bore me."

"Bore you?"

"I can't believe I'm saying that," he continued. "I have the perfect practice. I work with three other internal medicine doctors, and we rotate call, so that isn't even an issue anymore."

Hal paused for a moment, staring blankly out the window, and then continued. "I fight with myself, and then I just get more confused. I tell myself that life is good, but I don't really believe it. It's like I should be happy, but I'm not. I suppose everybody feels this way, but that doesn't help."

Hal shared about his practice, family and marriage, hobbies—which included biking and skiing—and church life. He was absolutely right:

It all sounded very nice. I too wondered why he was complaining. If anyone could claim to be normal, he could.

But then I saw it: Hal was living proof that normal and happy are not necessarily correlated. In fact, they often aren't. But I'm getting ahead of myself.

By the end of our first session I gave Hal an assignment. I asked him to carefully consider these questions and write out his responses:

1. What do you do for creative expression?

2. What do you do that others might consider edgy?

3. When do you feel most alive?

4. What risks do you take?

5. What barriers have you constructed that keep you from taking risks?

As you might imagine, Hal was stumped by several of my questions. In short, he did little to express his creativity. He did nothing others would consider edgy. Nothing came to mind when he thought about feeling most alive. He shared about taking a few risks on the slopes snow skiing, but even there he was cautious.

Hal's attention was piqued by the last question. In fact, he told me he was interested in the notion that perhaps he had constructed barriers to risk.

Mission accomplished. He was interested in taking the inner journey and was willing to look for ways he might be creating boredom in his life. In fact, he started thinking about the way being normal, or living nicely, might not always be a good thing.

By the end of our third session, Hal's demeanor had changed. He wasn't living any differently, but he had begun the journey we've talked about—the courageous inner journey. He was intrigued by the possibility that he had crafted a life exactly to his making and that it had become too nice. He had been coloring within the lines, allowing little room for imagination and growth.

Hal's healing would come only after some undoing. He needed to unravel the strands of his life that he had knitted too tightly together. His carefully regimented life gave little room for his spirit to breathe, so he started feeling bored and then depressed. He needed to take a journey into the wilder side of his personality, which he hadn't visited in years.

John the Baptist Wasn't Normal

Some parts of Scripture read like a Grisham story. We find thieves, murderers, tangled plots, and conspiracy. Just when you think you can predict the ending, in comes another terrorist, hero, or heroine. These passages certainly aren't tame. In fact, we wouldn't call very many people in the Bible normal.

John the Baptist was a prophet, but some people might have initially thought he was a lunatic. Here was a desert wanderer who called the religious leaders a brood of vipers. He pointed to a man who would come after him and be greater than him. He preached baptism of repentance for the forgiveness of sins. His message was strange and new. And if his message wasn't strange enough, consider his wardrobe and cuisine. Clothes of camel hair and a diet of locusts and wild honey.

John brought a message that was anything but normal. It eventually led to him being beheaded. Yet he lived his calling—to foretell the coming of the Messiah. He even had the incredible privilege of baptizing Jesus in the Jordan River.

Scripture is filled with stories of luminaries who sometimes seemed like lunatics.

Consider Daniel, another biblical character who refused to fit in. He had the wild idea of not defiling himself by eating the royal food, a plan that was sure to place him squarely in the face of danger. Fortunately, God had caused the official to show favor and sympathy to Daniel. Otherwise, the official would not have taken kindly to Daniel's idea of eating only vegetables and drinking water. Furthermore, Daniel had the audacity to challenge the official to test and see if Daniel didn't appear healthier than the young men who ate the royal food.

Fortunately, Daniel passed the test—and then some. "God gave [Daniel and his friends] knowledge and understanding of all kinds of literature and learning. And Daniel could understand visions and dreams of all kinds" (Daniel 1:17). Talk about creativity!

As the story unfolds, Daniel is able to interpret King Nebuchadnezzar's dreams (that's good). However, he predicts doom and gloom on the king (not so good). He and his friends refuse to pray to the king's gods and golden statue, so the king throws them into a furnace. Daniel later ignores King Darius' decree that prohibited prayer to anyone but the king, so the king throws him into a den of lions. The Lord protects him both times, but what an emotional price Daniel must have paid to follow his convictions!

Scriptures are replete with stories of men and women who acted out a calling that appeared to be anything but normal. Their lives included exciting, dramatic, and exhilarating episodes. The message to us is clear: Do we really want to be normal if normalcy means living safely and conforming to popular norms? Perhaps we need to rethink this whole idea of normalcy.

Barriers to Creativity, Imagination, and Freedom

Our consequences for living out our calling may not be as severe as Picasso's, John the Baptist's, or Daniel's, but still we are reluctant to express our unique talents, gifts, and creative expressions. We seem frozen in place, following the crowd. We feel a magnetic pull toward the center. Consider some of the many ways we're pulled into being average or normal.

1. We cling tenaciously to what we know. As if we were competing for a prize for holding on to familiarity for dear life, many of us plod through life, doing the same things day in and day out. We barely stop long enough to consider whether this is the life we really want to live.

We all know people who complain about their lives but cling fiercely to it. We ask them why, and they mutter a series of excuses. The truth is that they are familiar with their lives. They have them figured out. They know what to expect, and this brings a considerable sense of safety. But it often brings boredom and misery as well. Their lives lack freshness or spontaneity.

2. We cling to the familiar because we fear the unknown. Beneath our facade of acceptance is a terror of change. It is the rare Picasso, Daniel, or John the Baptist who is secure enough to swim upstream. We're all screaming, "Just let me blend in! I'll give anything to just blend in." And so we do. We buy a car like the neighbor's, live in a house like the neighbor's, go to a church like the neighbor's, and work in a business like the neighbor's. We not only want to keep up with the Joneses, we want to look just like them!

I've given examples of famous people whose individuality has been celebrated, but we know that things could go the other way. John the Baptist lost his head, Jesus was crucified, and many of our contemporaries have been ridiculed for their unique ideas.

3. We fear ridicule and judgment. Let's face it. A lot of people are ready to judge what they do not know. We settle into our known world because we're frightened of anyone who questions us. No one wants to face ridicule and contempt, and we know we will if we push boundaries.

Fortunately, we decide that forging our own trail is what we must do. We learn to endure a bit of rejection so we can go where we need to go. We learn to listen to our inner voice, stifling the outer voices. Being true to our inner voice, our true calling, will eventually be far more satisfying than following the masses.

4. We've been trained in conformity. We shouldn't be surprised that we value conformity. Our grade school teachers took over where our parents left off. We're supposed to look alike, think alike, work alike. For years we've been trained to conform. Why didn't we realize that the kids who got A's and the kids who got Fs got all the attention, while the rest of us sometimes got lost in the middle? Now that we look back, we can see that sometimes being average was worse than getting an F.

5. We've been trained to function on autopilot. For years we learned formulas, equations, and rules. And then we learned more rules. High marks were not given to the creative, but to the well-disciplined person with a fabulous memory and nice smile. Many of us developed a type of brain freeze. Paul Simon was right when he sang about all the stuff we learned in high school—it's a wonder we can think at all. The truth of the matter is, most of us don't think. We know what it takes to do our job well, and that's what we do. We know what it takes to fit in, and we do that. We know what it takes to earn a reasonable living— we don't even have to think anymore.

6. We've lacked opportunities for creative expression. I was raised in an era where a lot of men and some women worked at a job for 40 years, retired, got a gold watch, and moved to Arizona. Nothing was horrible about this life, but it certainly lacked creativity. Thousands upon thousands of Americans work for large corporations, take an early buyout, and fly to sunnier climes. Our Social Security system is built upon this notion. You work for 40 years, and we'll help you save a little so you might be able to enjoy lawn bowling and drive a golf cart around the complex. Again, this system isn't wrong, but it doesn't inspire creativity and fluid expression of interests.

Only in recent years have we heard about other options. As we boomers enter retirement, we are hearing about volunteer opportunities, classes we can take, languages we can learn, and hobbies we can take up. With medical advances being what they are and 60 years of age being more like what 45 was a few years ago, we've got some good options.

Taking Risks

Normal people don't take risks. OK, perhaps that's a bit dramatic, but there is certainly some truth in it.

While vacationing in Nerja, Spain, Christie and I met several American students from Middlebury, Vermont. They were studying abroad and had traveled from Granada to Málaga and up the coast to Nerja.

Talking with these kids was delightful. They had boundless energy, boundless enthusiasm, and a lifetime of boundless possibilities.

"Aren't you a bit nervous about traveling this far from home?" I asked.

Looking at me incredulously, a young man dressed in shorts, T-shirt, and sandals replied, "What do you mean?"

"Well, you're half a world away from home, away from everything and everyone you know, in an unfamiliar culture with an unfamiliar language. Isn't it a little weird?"

They looked at me calmly, and one replied. "No, not really. It takes some getting used to, but it's exciting. You have to let go of the familiar sometimes if you want to experience life."

I couldn't believe their maturity. As I continued to ask questions, I learned more about life, travel, and making adjustments than I could have from any book.

"How long will you be here?"

"We're on spring break from school and have to be back in Granada in a week."

"Was it hard at first to leave the U.S. and live in Spain?"

One of the girls responded, "Yeah, I had a tough time for the first few weeks over here. I miss some of my friends, my family, and the things I took for granted, like the Internet."

I smiled and nodded.

"We're addicted to the Internet, aren't we?"

"Not everyone in Europe," she answered, smiling. "We like things over here. There's a slower pace of life. And it's exciting. You just have to try new things sometimes."

We continued our conversation for several more minutes. Clearly these three students had become quite comfortable in this new world, far from their old, comfortable world in the United States, proving once again that we can push our boundaries and create a new sense of normal. But this involves risk.

Christie and I talked about these students as we walked back to our room. We noted that they had a self-confidence we certainly didn't have when we were their age. They were willing to take risks we never would have taken. They were willing to push the boundaries, perhaps even to the point of being considered abnormal. But they were having a ball doing it.

Remember Hal? His life was too nice. The antiseptic had leaked out of his consulting room into his life, creating a blanched existence. He and I spent many sessions exploring possibilities for his life. He was afraid something was wrong with him when his normal life no longer brought him joy.

As Hal explored what he might like to do, he realized he had limited himself to fitting into the normal mold. He became excited about changing and considering new possibilities. He had succeeded as a physician—what new mountains could he climb? What new horizons were calling his name? During our last session, he was considering a short-term mission into Central America with his wife. We'll see.

Latent Genius

Perhaps school and society have stifled the Picasso right out of you. Your Beethoven was squelched when your parents didn't recommend piano lessons. Your world of possibilities reached only to the edge of town, where you were strongly encouraged to stay. No full-ride scholarship to Princeton or Julliard.

Well, welcome to the club. We're all far more acquainted with no than we are with yes. We're accustomed to limits rather than possibilities. We know more about barriers than boundlessness. We see where we can't go rather than imagine where we can and must go. We're all part of the humongous bell-shaped curve called normal, which leaves our genius thirsty for expression. We've been dying to fit in, and now, before you know it, you are more normal than part of you wants to be. What to do now? That's the question.

As you continue on your journey, you may find yourself wanting to be a little less like everyone else. As you minimize your attempts to be normal and to conform, you may find that a little craziness may be what God has in mind for you. You may have a sudden urge to muss up your hair, fling open the patio doors, and belt out a song. You may start collecting the Sunday paper, circling cities in Europe you've secretly wanted to visit. You may have an incredible urge to walk into the boss' office and firmly say, "Thanks for this job. You can give it to someone else now."

These may not be your best options, though I'm excited if the Mozart or Michelangelo in you is stirring. But I've done part of my job if normalcy suddenly is not all it was cracked up to be. Perhaps a little Andy Warhol, Prince, or even Oprah isn't such a bad thing.

Do you have a latent genius? Are there areas of your life you've kept tamed all these years but are now ready to give a bit of breathing room? Can you imagine some small (maybe very small) ways you could experiment with zaniness?

Normalcy Revisited

As we navigate through this book, we must expand our thinking. I still firmly believe you're not as crazy as you think, but I want to get rid of the bell-shaped curve as your barometer for healthy living. I want to play with possibilities. I want you to push out the barriers you've defined as normal. I want you to consider that a little Picasso can be good for us.

Normal thinks like everyone else thinks.

Normal does what everyone else does.

Normal goes where everyone else goes.

Normal believes what everyone else believes.

Normal judges the way everyone else judges.

Does that still sound inviting? Are you sure you don't want just a hint of abnormalcy in your diet? Solomon said, "He has made everything beautiful in its time. He has also set eternity in the hearts of men" (Ecclesiastes 3:11). Might we have allowed ourselves to become too limited? We were created to be creative.

Perhaps we must redefine normalcy. We need to give more breathing room to the possibility of being normal and yet also creative. Imagine receiving compliments like these:

> That's crazy!
>
> You've got a wild imagination.
>
> What are you thinking?
>
> How could you do something like that?
>
> That's sure different than I'd do it.
>
> Are you sure you want to do that?
>
> Go for it!
>
> It's possible.

Now, imagine smiling back at them—those who are more bound by normalcy. Imagine having one foot in the camp of conformity and another in the zone of zaniness. Let's have a little fun with this stuff called normal. Let's hold the concept lightly in our hands while we proceed, exploring different ways we consider ourselves to be abnormal.

Lunatic or Visionary

As we think about Picasso, Daniel, John the Baptist, and Jesus, we must wrestle with the notions of lunatic and visionary. Picasso could see what others before him could not see. He learned what his teachers could teach him, and then he left them to forge his own trail. Certainly Jesus can be seen in the same light. Listen to words the prophet Isaiah spoke hundreds of years before Jesus' birth:

> He grew up before him like a tender shoot, and like a root out of dry ground. He had no beauty or majesty to attract us to him, nothing in his appearance that we should desire him. He was despised and rejected by men, a man of sorrows, and familiar with suffering. Like one from whom men hide their faces he was despised, and we esteemed him not (Isaiah 53:2-3).

The Jews sometimes accused Jesus of being demon possessed, but He was surely a visionary. Isaiah accurately foretold that Jesus would be Immanuel—God with us. He would come to save the people from their sins. Even now, lots of people aren't sure what to do with Jesus. They haven't decided for themselves whether He was crazy or whether He truly was and is the Messiah. But we know He came to shake up the world, to rattle the bones of the establishment. Surely Isaiah's prophecy was true:

> For to us a child is born, to us a son is given, and the government will be on his shoulders. And he will be called Wonderful Counselor, Mighty God, Prince of Peace. Of the increase of his government and peace there will be no end (Isaiah 9:6-7).

Having reconsidered this thing called normal, let's move forward and consider some of the many ways we feel abnormal and then look at some tools we can use to deal effectively with those feelings.

5

We're All
a Little Bit Nuts

*I remember when I used to sit on hospital
beds and hold people's hands, people used
to be shocked because they'd never seen this
before. To me it was quite normal.*

PRINCESS DIANA

We've come a long way in a few chapters. Have some of your nagging voices about craziness been silenced? Are you able to see some of the strengths hidden in some of your uniqueness?

The book began with a bold statement: We're all a little bit nuts. We're all a little bit crazy, and some of us are more crazy than others! We tend to feel abnormal, which leads to even greater feelings of anxiety and distress, so let's settle into the truth that we all have frayed places in our individual tapestry.

Remember the illustration of the mosaic—pieces of colored, broken, and misshapen glass jumbled into a beautiful work of art. Some pieces are light and airy; others are dark and distant. Some draw us to them, and others seem to repel us. All together, these pieces create magnificent images.

At times we don't feel like works of art, even though the psalmist David said you are fearfully and wonderfully made by the very hand of God, who knew you when you were being formed. Still, we feel broken, or misshapen, or odd. Rarely can we see from a distance how our pieces fit together to form something larger and grander than each individual piece.

Insecurity and anxiety are extremely uncomfortable emotions. With even a small amount of insecurity we feel as if we're coming apart at the seams. We question ourselves and wonder whether we're really all right or on the verge of losing control. Worse, we fear we might be losing our grip on reality.

But with a small dose of objectivity and reassurance that we're all a bit nuts, we can settle into our unique idiosyncrasies. Smiling as we embrace our peculiarities, we lovingly invite them closer, where we are open to what they might teach us. Becoming open and free, we can use our foibles to grow and become deeper, richer, and stronger people.

We have discovered that much of our distress comes from our secrecy and lack of objectivity. Fearing transparency—being vulnerable with others—we go into hiding. There, alone with our troubles, with myopic vision we amplify our problems and minimize others' difficulties. We imagine that everyone else's world is nice and tidy, and only our own marriage, family, and psyche are unraveling.

As you continue into your inner space discovery, you must be willing to face challenges and occasional danger. You've chosen to be brave; now you'll also need to be curious and learn to decipher code. You must be able to live with uncertainty. What else can you realistically do when you meet alienated thoughts and feelings and distorted images? In daydreams, night dreams, and the simple musings of everyday life, inner space requires you to set aside judgments and preconceptions. But inner space travel is necessary if you really want to embrace your individuality and regain a sense of normalcy.

The Journey Toward Normal

With all the push to be normal and the incessant clamoring to fit in, we lose something. We want to be normal and fit in, but we also must maintain and sometimes regain our individuality. We want to embrace the excitement we feel when striking out on our own journey—our unique course.

Normalcy, remember, is not helpful when it means living up to another's standards or conforming to another's rules for living. We too easily surrender our novel ideas to the ideas of the group. We relinquish dreams in favor of group consensus. This feels devastating. What if your standards are not mine? What if your rules for conformity hem me in?

Remember Cassandra, the pastor's wife who felt so guilty? She wasn't willing to conform to unrealistic expectations of how she should live as the pastor's wife. She was considering following her own path in worship and ministry.

How about Hal, the physician whose life was so sanitized that it was becoming mind-numbingly boring? His antiseptic world had no room for wildness.

Both Cassandra and Hal lost touch with their true self as they tried to squeeze into the mold of who they were expected to be. Each lost the juice that comes from living close to their creative self. Feelings of craziness, we saw, often come from losing touch with what is important to us. Trying to be square pegs in round holes was driving Cassandra and Hal crazy.

Did I tempt you at all by the stories of Picasso, Daniel, or John the Baptist? They would never be described as being average. Does the craziness of Leonardo da Vinci ever appear exciting to you? Do you ever want to throw caution to the wind and try something new, extravagant, wild?

When I think of anyone who has made a distinct mark on the world—Columbus, Rembrandt, Shakespeare, or even Steven Spielberg, I'm aware of how different he or she is. Those people didn't readily fit in. They stretched the limits and risked being considered a lunatic. They took incredible chances, often raising eyebrows and criticism. But in the end, we called them geniuses.

Dancing with Normal

As we discovered in chapter 2, we have a push-pull relationship with the whole concept of normalcy. On the one hand, we idolize people who are willing to stick their necks out and succeed. Who ever imagined a person would start a company like eBay and revolutionize the way we buy things? Or create a company like Google and create such a change in the way we seek information that the word has become a recognizable verb! I google a lot when I'm writing.

Conversely, we often frown on rebels who try and fail. We speak disparagingly of people who had a wild idea and landed facedown on the pavement. The ridicule they experience too often frightens us from attempting something new.

We want to retain our sense of individuality, so we search out comparisons to confirm we're not as different from others as we sometimes feel. We want to feel normal. Still, we don't want to be hemmed in by others' expectations of us. See what I mean? Push-pull.

The key, it seems—and this is critical—is not to get too concerned about being normal. We must not become so engrossed with being normal that everything we think, feel, and do serves that end. We dare not believe that because something is normal, it is right for us. We don't always have to be average, though we usually are.

At the other extreme, completely disregarding what most others do isn't helpful either. We want to develop an easy alliance with this notion. We want to dance lightly with the concept of normalcy.

Again, the trick is to consider what others do, how they live, and what they think, but not to let those things control us. In some cases you'll be influenced by others, allowing them to impact and change you. In other circumstances, what they think won't matter to you. Finding the right balance is sometimes difficult.

How can we dance lightly with differing interests? We dance lightly by fully appreciating that the range of normalcy is wide indeed. We're music aficionados ranging from opera to Dave Mathews; we're artists ranging from Matisse to paint by number; we're writers ranging from esoteric poetry to Hemingway to Louis L'Amour. With an open heart, we explore all of our thoughts and feelings, giving room for their expression even if they don't seem normal at first glance.

How do we dance lightly with idiosyncrasies? We dance lightly by withholding quick judgments about ourselves and others. We prefer things to be a certain way, but that doesn't mean they must be so. We prefer certain character traits, but that doesn't give us a right to dictate their existence. You'll see how this unfolds as we talk about specific character traits.

Redefining Idiosyncrasies

We casually use the phrase *a little bit nuts,* but for many this colloquialism carries genuine angst. Many are painfully aware of the ways they don't fit in and quickly label their behavior as abnormal. This labeling increases their anxiety. No one wants to feel crazy.

We must remember that everyone has some rough edges. Many have challenging relationships with one or both parents, and nearly everyone can cite some place in his childhood where things could have been much better. Everyone has had a relationship turn sour and has wondered what role she played in the mess. Everyone has been accused of wrongdoing and has known in his heart that some of the blame lies squarely at his feet.

As we begin to explore some of our common problems and idiosyncrasies, we must remember that courageous exploration provides opportunities for growth. Every wound is a place where we can become stronger. Every idiosyncrasy is a challenge for us to be honest with ourselves about the true extent of our foibles.

For example, I tend to want things to be structured. I dislike chaos, and frenetic environments make me uncomfortable. I can structure my own surroundings without causing problems for me or others. But when I drift into structuring others' lives or environments, I violate their boundaries, and nobody likes that.

I also have a low tolerance for family chaos and drama. Consequently,

I've been accused of being too detached from my family of origin. My parents would like us to gather with my extended family—three sisters, a brother, and their mates—every other week. Once every six weeks is plenty for me. You can imagine some of the criticism Christie and I receive for living three hours away and being available so infrequently.

We all have habits that range from being a nuisance to being downright annoying. I know this because we're all a little bit nuts. You have habits, traits, and idiosyncrasies that can cause more than a little havoc. We're going to take a look at some of our habits. But first, let's remind ourselves of where they came from.

It All Began When...

None of us came from perfect parents, so we shouldn't expect to be perfect ourselves. In fact, no child will grow up without a few scars. I've seen good parents do damage to children. I've also seen bad parents do horrendous damage to children. I've also witnessed terrible parents do wonderful things for their children. Parenting, as James Dobson says, isn't for cowards.

I'm always amazed that any parent can raise a healthy child, given the obstacles to parenting. Most children are born into families with much love. But unfortunately, love is not enough, and the many pitfalls that fall on adults trickle down to the innocent children.

This is not to trivialize childhood trauma. Children should be raised in an atmosphere of innocence and profound respect, but that ideal is rarely realized. Abuse happens; some parents are neglectful and abandon their children. In fact, many parents lose their parental rights because they have been abusive.

Perhaps parents' primary challenge is to raise children who learn to function effectively in their adult world. We're proud if our children navigate their way through the multitude of childhood problems and become healthy adults. But unfortunately, many times growth is deterred, and troublesome traits develop. We can easily stray from developing into normal, healthy adults and become abnormal unhealthy adults. Let's look at some of the common places where detours occur.

Common Detours

None of us are perfect. Even with the best childhood, many develop character traits that are within the range of normalcy but are nonetheless unhealthy. I have identified eight common traits that can range from slightly annoying to downright dysfunctional, depending on their severity.

These eight prevalent traits show up again and again in my clinical practice. They cause significant worry for the individual or for his or her family. All of these traits are quite common, and I wouldn't be surprised if you recognize yourself in some of them. As we explore them, ask yourself to what extent you exhibit these behaviors.

Pretension

Picture a couple of four-year-olds playing together. Each feels she is the center of the universe. You hear one say, "Look at me," but the other barely notices. In fact, she shows off even more.

Watch and listen closely, and you'll notice that the two children want to control their toys, their play, and even the way the other behaves. You'll hear, "Don't do it that way," "No," or "Stop it." These children behave with more than a small dose of egocentricity, they are obsessed with their world, and they don't care how their behavior impacts others.

We expect this self-centered posturing in children. We expect them to act like kings or queens of the castle, and in some ways we teach them that they are. In time, however, we want them to become socialized and to care about others' feelings and lives.

Troubles will occur if this pretension doesn't fade and create room for more mature thoughts and actions, such as sensitivity, mutuality, and consideration. The troubles might include legal transgressions, work issues, and most certainly, relationship difficulties. A person who hasn't learned that the world doesn't revolve around him is not fun to be with for more than a few minutes.

We all have the capacity to be pretentious and arrogant, but when this trait grows from a small dose into a huge dollop, you're in danger. Pretension pushes people away. Arrogance leaves little room for others to share their feelings, thoughts, or concerns. It leaves little room for the mature trait of mutuality.

The apostle Paul says it like this: "Do not think of yourself more highly than you ought, but rather think of yourself with sober judgment, in accordance with the measure of faith God has given you" (Romans 12:3). The message is clear—you're no better or worse than anybody else. We're all in this boat together!

Possessiveness

These same four-year-old children struggle to share anything. When one of them touches something that belongs to the other, you may hear a bloodcurdling screech: "That's mine! Give it back!"

A skirmish breaks out quickly as each child tugs at the desired toy. A push here, a shove there. They may even resort to heavy-handed tactics like biting—all because of a toy they want.

This trait is also normal and to be expected in children. Children naturally believe the world revolves around them, and anything they can reach is theirs. This is a normal stage for children to pass through.

When we watch typical four-year-olds at play, we quickly see their propensity to hoard what they believe belongs to them. Helpful parents take this behavior to heart and recognize that relationships falter when people don't learn the art of sharing.

In the delightful book *All I Really Need to Know I Learned in Kindergarten*, Robert Fulghum counts sharing as one of the basic traits people need for successful development. He notes that this is so basic that one would think it hardly needs mentioning. However, a glance at many adult relationships, some in serious trouble, often reveals that the parties are hooked in power struggles, each person wanting his own way. They demand that others agree with them; they insist things go their way. Instead of an attitude of giving and generosity, they're caught in possessiveness. You can almost hear their childish voices saying, "Give it back. It's mine. This is the way I do it."

Personalizing

At the slightest disappointment, many young children will scream, rant, and rave. If their ice-cream cone drops on the floor, you'd think their world was coming to an end. Their histrionics are notorious. Every mole-hill becomes a mountain, and parents scramble to calm them down.

Children have little ability to tolerate frustration. They seem to be saying, "Don't disappoint me. I can't stand it," or "I can't stand this." When things don't go their way, they're quick to feel as if someone is waging a personal assault against them. Being egocentric, they take rejection personally.

Youngsters naturally and normally personalize events, but as we mature, we learn to see beyond the immediate situation. Your parents, for example, didn't set out to reject or abandon you. They didn't plot to create a hostile environment. It's not all about you! They were caught up in their own lives, and you suffered some of the consequences.

To feel the sting of rejection or to hurt when things don't go your way is normal, but you will respond in a healthier way when you remember that the events that unfolded didn't conspire against you. Sometimes stuff just happens.

Pathologizing

When our four-year-old experiences the slightest frustration, she can be devastated. A broken toy or a postponed trip to the zoo can make her feel as if her world is caving in. She turns the incident into a disease and thinks, *Bad things always happen to me* or *Nothing ever goes my way.* She quickly imagines the worst-case scenario.

We've all pathologized our troubles at times. We've all endured a series of unfortunate events and felt like the little boy Judith Viorst described in *Alexander and the Terrible, Horrible, No Good, Very Bad Day*. But as adults, we know that one bad day doesn't predict the next. Temporary experiences can paint a gloomy canvas, and that's normal, but a healthier response is to put things in perspective. Things will look brighter in the morning. Truth be told, you've probably had more fortunate occurrences than unfortunate ones. It's all a matter of which ones get the most attention.

Playing the Victim

A close cousin to pathologizing is playing the victim. Imagine two more four-year-olds at play, and one is a whiner. The whiner has already begun to see the dark side of every situation. He feels that things never work out his way and that he always gets the worst of the deal. More important, this child feels he's done nothing wrong to deserve the treatment he's getting. He's innocent, and someone else is always to blame for his plight.

This too is a childish trait that many adults have elevated to a fine art. Every troubling event makes them think, *Poor me*. Perhaps you've been around people who cannot see the good events in their lives because they're so focused on the bad. Attempts to cheer them up are in vain—they absorb all your energy if you try to fix them.

Even when they cause their own trouble, these victims have a way of turning things into someone else's fault. They want you to feel sorry for them. This common trait is obviously very damaging to adult relationships. Instead of taking responsibility for their problems, victims twist and distort events so they are the innocent of someone else's dastardly deeds. Interacting with someone so childish can be incredibly frustrating.

Perfectionism

Imagine two more four-year-olds playing a game. One has learned how to take charge, lining up the toys the way she says is right and insisting on a certain way to play. There are rules to be followed, she asserts. She doesn't notice that the other has her own way of playing or ignores her playmate's protests. Can you imagine the trouble that is brewing? The queen watches her friend like a hawk, ready to pounce on her for infractions. She has a rigid way of expecting things to be.

Her friend has few choices. She can go along with the controller, she can attempt to assert her power, or she can quit the game—which most often occurs. Soon the game is no game at all, but a series of strategic moves as each child criticizes the other until one of them finally quits.

Perfectionism doesn't work in adult life either. In fact, to live with criticism is to flounder in a sea of rights and wrongs, always feeling on the wrong end of things.

We know the feeling of being controlled. It is painful and discouraging. How must people feel when they continue their demanding ways into adulthood? They live in a restrictive world of right and wrong, black and white. Their eye is quickly drawn to what isn't perfect—the dishes left on the counter, the dirty clothes hanging out of the hamper, and the dust that has collected on the piano. Their work is never done.

To want order in our lives and to live by some rules is natural and normal, but sometimes we need to let things flow. Easy does it. We need time to play, just as we need time to work. Sometimes we need to bend the rules, and sometimes we need order.

You can guess where normalcy turns into obsessive-compulsive disorder or where perfectionism becomes control. To run your own world by a rigid set of rights and wrongs is one thing; to impose those standards on others is something else entirely. On the other side of the coin, for laid-back people to let their old newspapers stack up by the easy chair is one thing; to refuse to dispose of them is quite another. A normal, natural tendency can easily become a bone of contention.

Passive-Aggressive Behavior

We all express anger and aggression, and we do it in direct, healthy ways or indirect, unhealthy ways. Imagine children who are angry with one another but haven't a clue how to express that anger in a direct and healthy manner. What might they do to express their anger indirectly?

Children can be sarcastic, put down their friends' ideas, or refuse to play with them. They commonly pout, ignore one another, or even destroy their friends' belongings. All these are ways of seeking revenge on others for hurting them.

Many adults still cling to these childish behaviors because they don't know how to express anger and displeasure in healthy ways. When conflicts arise—and they will—healthy people learn to sit down, look their partner in the eye, and discuss differences and solutions. But this rarely occurs. More often than not, people are prone to hold grudges, "forget" important matters, pout, or make sarcastic comments. All these options erode the warmth and affection of a relationship.

Anger is normal. Sniping at your mate on occasion is typical. But allowing passive-aggressive behaviors to rule your relationship is unhealthy. We must learn to deal with aggression in direct, honest, and compassionate ways.

Pugnacity

Even preschools have bullies. Some children are ready to fight, to use aggression to get what they want. Whether they are bigger, stronger, or simply more willful, some children will use sheer force to get what they want, pushing, shoving, and calling names. They don't care how their behavior makes others feel.

Tyrants in the adult world refuse to harness their aggression, favoring instead occasional bouts of bluster. Childish temper tantrums remain in many adult relationships.

When we threw tantrums as children, we were sent to our rooms, given a chance to cool down, and told that these displays of aggression would not be allowed. We were socialized. But some of us didn't learn our lessons. We've taken our pugnacity into our adult lives and continued to bully people around. A bit of this trait makes for strong leadership, so we shouldn't be surprised to find this quality in the leaders of many corporations, courtrooms, and other organizations.

Pugnacity runs out of grace at some point. People tire of walking on eggshells around forceful, tyrannical brutes. We steer clear of them. If we are married to them, we tend to push away emotionally and physically unless they change their ways.

Adjustment

Healthy adults adjust to adversity. We give up childish traits for the good of effective adult relationships. Traumatic experiences often throw us off course, but we should expect that. If you experienced childhood trauma, your development was forever altered. If you slipped into addictions in adolescence and are only now recovering, your life trajectory has been forever changed. But don't lose heart. It's never too late to grow up.

The question isn't how badly you've been hurt or how much you've lost to your addiction. Rather, what are you doing right now to facilitate your recovery? Are you focusing your energies on growing, healing, improving, and learning?

Cami is a 24-year-old woman with three young children who were fathered by three different men. Raised in a broken and dysfunctional family, Cami learned to fend for herself, albeit poorly. She grew into a hardened adolescent and was attracted to boys who were as troubled as she was. She was buried in a life of drugs and alcohol, and the last six years of her life are a blur. Appearing thin and tired, she came to me because of her feelings of depression.

Cami was struggling financially and raising her children as a single mother, but amazingly, she still had a spark in her eyes. She had just finished drug and alcohol treatment and wanted to come to terms with her painful childhood. She wanted to understand how her early years of neglect, which left her with few healthy models of how to survive in an adult world, was impacting her life now.

Cami is starting to develop some goals for her life. Previously she lived for one day and possibly the next, but never for the future. Now she wants to dream a little. She is considering being a pediatric nurse so she can help other children who have been abused.

"I know what it feels like to be moved from foster home to foster home," she said sadly, looking away as she began to cry. "I don't think any child should have to live like that. No one seemed to care about me. I want to be a nurse to show children that someone cares about how they are doing and will help them feel better."

"Why did you have to go to foster homes?" I asked.

"My mom and dad are losers," she continued. "Both are still into drugs. Dad hasn't worked for years, and I don't know what my mom is doing. I want to figure out who I am."

"How did you become such a survivor?" I asked. "You have three children, and you're working on going to college—that's pretty impressive."

"Sometimes I don't think I can make it," she admitted. "Believe me, I get really discouraged. But I have some friends at church who encourage me. An older couple from church watches the kids when I'm in school, and they're like the parents I never had."

"They sound wonderful."

"They are wonderful. They're giving me a new chance. They show me God's love."

"Do you ever feel like giving up?"

"Yeah, I do. I wish I could just stay home with the kids. They're growing up without me a lot. I work and go to school, and they miss me. It makes me sad."

"But you have a plan?" I asked.

"Sort of. I'm not sure of myself. What I know is that I can't slip back into using drugs and drinking. That got me nowhere. My kids need a good home, and I've got some friends who are willing to help."

Cami appeared sad, but she spoke with determination.

"I could sit home and watch television. I've been there and done that. That only made me more depressed. I don't want to be a victim any more. I felt sorry for myself for a long time, and that didn't really help. Now I know that I'm the only one who can make things better for the kids. I thank God for His love and for bringing some wonderful people into my life."

Cami had a glow in her eyes when she talked about her dreams. She's lived many lifetimes in her 24 years. She's gained a perspective that is helping her. She can do with her life as she chooses.

Cami is a model for all of us. She's lived beyond adversity. Previously stuck being a victim, she now chooses to live up to her full potential. She still struggles with periods of discouragement, but she's pushing forward.

Getting Stuck in Your Childhood

Childhood is a breeding ground for all sorts of problems. Children lack the skills to transform these normal but destructive traits into socialized and constructive behavior. That's where parents come in. Many of our issues start out as normal childhood traits but then turn into niggling adult character problems. We need to keep from getting stuck in these problems.

Dr. Laura Schlessinger, in her book *Bad Childhood, Good Life,* says, "Many folks just stay stuck in their childhood ugliness—for decades, sometimes forever, angry, bitter, self-destructive, depressed, anxious, or just generally out of control and way off any positive track."[1]

Schlessinger is an optimist about moving beyond childhood difficulties. (I am too.) She believes in the indomitable spirit of people. She carefully makes a distinction between people *with* a past and people who are *defined* by their past. This is a very useful way of thinking about our difficulties.

People *with* a past understand the influences parents and others have had on their lives. They've worked with those influences and not allowed them to control their lives. People *defined* by their past tend to cling to their early childhood wounds, building their sense of identity around what's happened to them. Dr. Schlessinger goes on to offer this encouragement:

When your early life is basically one threat after another to your sanity and physical self, it's hard not to "live in your feelings." Unfortunately, that can get to be a way of life that precludes growth and joy, which generally come from attention to others than yourself.[2]

Review the list of childish Ps and put them in perspective. Can you see them as idiosyncrasies that need attention but that don't define you? This is critical. Can you see you are not a product of your experiences, but of your ongoing response to those experiences?

- Consider moving from possessiveness to generosity. When you have the choice, share.

- Consider moving from personalizing difficulties to understanding that things often unfold randomly. Also consider seeing your role in whatever might be occurring in your life and focusing on changing it.

- Consider moving from pathologizing to putting issues in perspective. This too shall pass. Your life is filled with blessings as well as challenges. You can determine how to solve the problems facing you.

- Consider moving from playing the victim to taking responsibility. No one wants to be around a martyr. People gravitate toward people who are responsible.

- Consider giving up perfectionism and living with more grace. Rigidity, along with right-and-wrong thinking, hems people in and pushes them away from you. Perfectionism restricts you and inhibits possibilities.

- Consider giving up passive-aggressive behavior, moving toward healthy expression of anger. Learn to share your feelings, expressing specifically what you want and need from others.

- Consider giving up pugnacity, moving instead toward respect for others. Determine never to disrespect others with your bullying tendencies. Always respect other people's boundaries.

This is quite a substantial list, but it catapults us beyond being stuck in childhood into healthy adult living. Maybe you were victimized. Maybe you were raised with violence, rejection, or outright abandonment. We all have childhood trauma—some of us more than others. We've all had setbacks from divorce, death, financial ruin, or some other calamity. *That's normal.* What are you doing about it now? That is the primary question. You may have had a bad childhood, but that doesn't mean you can't have a wonderful life now.

Embracing Your Challenges

Do you understand where normal ends and unhealthiness begins? Can you see childhood patterns of behavior that are perfectly normal but that become unhealthy when they continue into adulthood?

In this chapter you learned about the dance of self-acceptance on the one hand and growth on the other. The apostle Paul writes about running the race even when it's difficult. Listen to his words.

> Do you not know that in a race all the runners run, but only one gets the prize? Run in such a way as to get the prize. Everyone who competes in the games goes into strict training. They do it to get a crown that will not last; but we do it to get a crown that will last forever. Therefore I do not run like a man running aimlessly; I do not fight like a man beating the air. No, I beat my body and make it my slave so that after I have preached to others, I myself will not be disqualified for the prize (1 Corinthians 9:24-27).

> I press on to take hold of that for which Christ Jesus took hold of me. Brothers, I do not consider myself yet to have taken hold of it. But one thing I do: Forgetting what is behind and straining toward what is ahead, I press on toward the goal

to win the prize for which God has called me heavenward
in Christ Jesus (Philippians 3:12-13).

For we are God's workmanship, created in Christ Jesus to
do good works, which God prepared in advance for us to
do (Ephesians 2:10).

We are being changed from the inside out—thank God! And we
are not only growing up but also being prepared for good works. You
have a challenge facing you, a specific purpose for which God has gifted
you. Can you embrace the challenge of moving beyond unhelpful
normal behavior patterns into maturity? Can you allow God to work
in you, perfecting you for His purpose?

We're all a little bit nuts. We all have traits that cause challenges in
our life. We see them, we experience them, and now we can choose to
cooperate with God as He transforms them.

In our next chapter we'll explore our tendency to believe everyone
is talking about us—or that they would if we exposed some of our
vulnerabilities. We'll see how to face these beliefs, embrace them, and
change them.

6

Everybody's Talkin' About Me

*We wouldn't worry so much about what people think
of us if we knew how seldom they do.*

Try as I might to dispel the feeling, at times I still think people are talking about me. Don't get me wrong—I'm not paranoid, I don't hear voices, and I have never thought people were out to get me. Still, after I've left a room or said something I thought was particularly humorous or stupid, I'm afraid people talk about me. I imagine them saying, "David thinks he's so funny when he's not." I want them to say, "He's hilarious!"

I know I'm not alone. Perhaps you share the same concern. Maybe you struggle with opening your mouth in public because you're afraid someone might have negative thoughts about you. Or perhaps recently you've been at a party and wondered just what people thought of you.

Well, join the crowd. Being afraid of what people think of us is one of our most common fears, right behind public speaking. We all worry about what others might think of us. Sometimes our concern can be paralyzing.

Melody Beattie is a household name in the addiction's recovery movement. Pioneering much of what we understand about codependency, she has written numerous bestsellers, including her seminal work *Codependent No More*. The book touched a chord in people. Many people raised in alcoholic families quickly identified with the desire to please others at their own expense. They identified with Beattie's observations that individuals raised in dysfunctional families had a fractured sense of self. Codependents, as people pleasers are called, derive their self-esteem from what others think about them rather than from their own sense of well-being.

Beattie's theories spread like wildfire beyond the field of drug and alcohol recovery into the mainstream. Soon, other people—folks who weren't raised in alcoholic or drug-involved homes—related to her ideas about codependency. She proclaimed that people could be raised in healthy, middle-class families, attend church twice on Sunday, and still be codependent.

Soon other pioneers joined her, like Pia Mellody and John Bradshaw. They spoke about the loss of self and the desire to live from the outside in rather than from the inside out. They highlighted the likelihood that we will live according to the expectations of others rather than be true to our own values.

Thoroughly appreciating their work, I wrote *When Pleasing Others Is Hurting You,* which also found a receptive audience. Christians, it seemed, also struggled with hypersensitivity to what others said about them. I wrote about our twisted notion of feeling somehow more pious (but also lost and depressed) when we give and give and give regardless of what happens to us and our families. We are confused about what losing our lives for the sake of the gospel means.

Tuned into the opinions of others, we look to them for our bearings, and we easily become lost. Plotting our course solely on the counsel of others leaves us vulnerable and often confused. Turning exclusively to others for our direction is like setting our compass a few degrees off. Who knows where we might end up?

The Thin Line of Approval

Nobody likes to be around narcissists, who live and breathe for their own opinions and perceptions. Narcissists believe the world revolves around them. They are self-centered and myopic, often controlling, and difficult to live with. They don't care about your opinion and aren't likely to ask for it. They couldn't care less about your point of view.

Although I am not promoting this immature perspective, the opposite side of the coin—caring too much about others' opinions—isn't any healthier. A thin line separates an appropriate sensitivity to others from a crippling need for their approval. As you become better equipped to discern the difference, you notice the value of listening to others without allowing them to direct your life.

Most of us are overly sensitive about others' opinions, and this sensitivity drives us nuts. With a huge desire to please, we don't just want to know what others think; we want their approval. Lacking a clear sense of our own identity, we beg others to approve of what we think, feel, and want. We barely take a step without checking it out with someone whose approval we desire. This creates a feeling of chaos and craziness inside us.

Consider the difference between wanting approval and needing approval. Most of us want others to approve of what we're doing. We take some pleasure in knowing that the people who are important to us—our parents, friends, and mate—agree with what we're doing with our lives. This is normal and natural.

But what if we *need* the approval of others? What if we can't make a decision unless the people who are important to us approve of what we're doing? You can imagine how quickly our lives become small and restricted. We're handcuffed and taken hostage by a few people's opinions. We give those people enormous power to direct our lives.

I'm an admitted card-carrying codependent—in recovery. I've lived many of my 56 years of life needing other people's approval. I'm growing beyond this childish behavior. I'm thinking for myself, making decisions on my own, and taking some chances. I still care what others think, but I'm not driven by their approval.

As I write this chapter, I'm purchasing a sailboat. This may not seem like a big deal, but it seems to be a big deal to a lot of people in my world. Many disapprove of the purchase.

"Why do you want to own a boat when you can rent one for a fraction of the price? Think it over," the marina manager said the other day, with a disapproving scowl on his face.

"Are you sure you know what you're doing?" my dad asked not long ago, with his fatherly, opinionated tone. "You know a boat is a hole in the water you throw money into."

"Are you going to use it enough to warrant the expense?" a friend asked.

Everyone I talked to seemed critical of my sailboat idea, causing me to second-guess my decision. The more input I received, the more confused I felt. I felt irritated and sat down with Christie so she could help me sort out my feelings.

"I get annoyed at what everyone is saying to me about the boat purchase," I said with obvious frustration. "I thought I knew what I was doing, but now I'm not so sure."

"David," Christie said with concern, "you listen to all those people. You let them influence you. In some cases you ask for their opinion."

"But I don't want their criticism and discouragement," I replied. "I care what everybody thinks."

"If you need their approval, then don't get the boat," she said, smiling, with more than a hint of sarcasm.

OK. That caught my attention. Good point. If I really *need* their approval, I'll forget about the boat, put my money into a certificate of deposit at the bank, and stop my dreamy musing about sailing the Puget Sound waters.

What if my conversation with my dad had unfolded like this?

"David," my dad might say, "I really think you need to reconsider buying that sailboat. Your mother and I have been talking. You're only going to use it three, maybe four months of the year. It's got a lot of wood on it, and that takes a lot of upkeep. The sails will need tending to and the motor must be kept up. The whole thing will take time away from you and your marriage. You don't want that to happen, do you?"

I care about my parents' opinion, so I'd be reconsidering the whole situation, to be sure. But that wouldn't end my problems because I still want the boat!

Thankfully, I don't need their approval. I'd like it but don't need it. As part of my recovery from codependence, I'm being more cautious about whom I talk about important issues in my life with. I also remind myself that not everyone will approve of my decisions, and that's OK.

Thrown off Balance

Being sensitive to the opinions of others, some of us are easily thrown off course. Our grasp on our reality seems tenuous, and if we know others are talking about us and disapproving of us, we're in for a tough time.

I've been working with a 50-year-old woman named Kelly. She's had a rough life, and her wrinkled skin suggests years of smoking and perhaps excessive drinking. Divorced twice, Kelly feels sad about the losses she's experienced in each of these marriages.

Kelly is a thin, wispy woman with two grown children. She doesn't laugh easily, she complains of feeling depressed at times, and she says she is discouraged about her past and her future. For more than two years, I've been walking with her through her second divorce and helping her settle into her single life.

Kelly has been depressed most of her adult life. She married men who were either alcoholic or chronically angry, so she's felt her share of sadness, abandonment, and loss. She feels a keen sense of having missed out on a life of her own.

Kelly is also enmeshed with her demanding mother. Her mother is single as well, and now that Kelly is single, her mother feels even more entitled to make demands on Kelly. Kelly finds this hard to refuse.

In spite of her depressive and often angry tones, Kelly has found a new spark of life since divorcing her angry, bitter, and abusive husband. She works as an attorney and has found satisfaction again in her work. She seems to be breathing a bit easier.

Recently Kelly announced she's planning to move to California to live near her sister, with whom she has a close and supportive relationship. Though this idea has been gurgling inside her for many months, she is just now talking seriously about it.

"My mother doesn't like the idea. She thinks I'm nuts. My siblings don't like the idea either, but then why would they? I'm the one watching out for Mom. They're all talking about me, thinking I'm deserting her. Somehow I got appointed to make sure everything goes OK for her."

"How did you get that job?" I asked.

"I've always had it," she said sadly. "I'm a natural caretaker. I did it with the men in my life, and I do it with my mom. I can't seem to help it. I've always been close to my mom, and sometimes I've actually enjoyed being her caretaker. But now I hate how much she's grown to lean on me. I want to move to California, where the weather will be better and where I can be close to my sister. I feel like I need more freedom."

"Sounds great, Kelly. What's stopping you?"

"I know the whole family thinks I'm going off the deep end," she said. "I've got a thriving practice. Getting another practice going in California would take some work. They all think I'm nuts."

"What do you think?" I asked.

"I think I want to take a chance," she chuckled. "Why not? I'm single. I can sell my house and get a smaller one in California. I don't need so much room. I'll be close enough to drive or fly up to see my kids. This feels like a good time to make a change."

"Listen to how clear you are, Kelly."

"Well, I am clear," she said, her voice trailing off. "But my family doesn't approve. My mom hates the idea. My brothers and sisters are against it. Even my colleagues have cautioned me about the challenges of starting up a new practice at my age. I've been rethinking my decision."

Kelly is understandably ambivalent. She feels confused as she listens to many different voices giving her contrary advice. That's the problem with getting too much counsel or listening to too many voices—we lose our own vision.

Unwanted Advice

We've all had people tell us what we should do, what we should feel, and how we should change our lives. Everybody has an opinion. With all these people clamoring about what is best for us, hearing our own inner voice can be difficult.

Kelly's problem with unwanted advice has been termed *emotional incest* by some psychologists. These experts believe that when others tell us what to do or how to do it, they violate us in a most basic way. They commit the emotional equivalent of jumping over your fence and robbing you.

Most of us are too polite to say anything, but inside we feel this violation. We know that some of our closest friends and our dearest family members are talking about us. Some have the audacity to tell us to our face that they're talking about us! We feel the violation. We sense the robbery of something dear to us: our right to think what we think, feel what we feel, make the decisions we want to make, and accept responsibility for those choices.

Though frightened to say it, we want to scream out, "Let me live my own life! I know what's best for me, and this is what I want to do. Even if I make some mistakes, they're my mistakes. Leave me alone."

But we don't scream out. We wince, and our stomachs wrench from resentment. Our heads ache as we try to process the controlling and often conflicting messages coming at us. We know we don't like to be patronized, but we don't know what to do about it.

Kelly shared a recent conversation with her mother.

"My mom told me I really shouldn't move. She said, 'It's so hot in California and so incredibly busy. There are wall-to-wall people. You won't have the freedom you have here in Washington.'"

"Your mom knows what's best for you?" I asked sarcastically. "She is able to read into your future and know what you should do with your life? I don't think so."

"She's always had an opinion about my life. She always knows what's best for me. I used to buy it wholesale, but now it just makes me angry."

"It is awfully presumptuous when you think about it," I said. "Your mom talks like she knows you and what's best for you. I get annoyed when someone has the audacity to tell me what to do without my permission."

Kelly seemed a bit startled by that.

"I guess I've always thought I should listen to my mom, as if it was the Christian thing to do. Now I know that's not true."

One of the vestiges of my own codependency has been the tendency to ask too many people for too much advice—and then to try to listen to all of it. When making the decision on the sailboat, I asked no fewer than 20 people what they thought of my idea. You might laugh at my insecurity, and rightly so. I'm working on that.

You might also understand the pure nonsense of getting so much counsel. To seek advice can be a good thing. But to ask someone to make your decisions for you or to try to manipulate your friends into understanding your thoughts and feelings is not. Too much counsel can be a bad thing indeed, and I'm learning to tone it down.

Kelly and I talked about her tendency to share her precious ideas with too many people—especially those who do not treat them with respect. We worked on setting firmer boundaries and having the courage to follow her dreams.

Clearly, too many people ask too many other people for too much advice. We get as many opinions as the number of people we ask, so of course we end up feeling alone and thinking, *Huh?*

People are eager to give their opinions. They tell us what they think we should do. We must remember it is really impossible for others to accurately tell us what we should do, even though they'd like to. They don't know our innermost feelings. They don't know what is acutely important to us. The best they can do is offer opinions from their vantage point, which has obvious limitations. Should we be surprised that we're confused?

People will quickly offer opinions about our lives, and this is usually very annoying, but we must look inside for the problem. They may be ready to give us answers to our problems and advice to our concerns, but we rarely stop them! We listen to them talk and talk and talk as our brains become more and more muddled.

I worked with Kelly to turn down the volume on her siblings' advice. I encouraged her to stop sharing so much of her plan with people who stomped on it. These dreams and goals, we agreed, were precious, tiny seeds that need just the right soil and sunlight to germinate. They wouldn't grow in a hostile environment.

Another way to consider Kelly's problems, and perhaps your own, is to use the language of boundaries. We don't have to feel compelled to share our dreams with everyone. We can carefully choose the people we seek advice from or share our dreams with. In fact, good boundaries dictate that we consider where and when to share what is important to us. Even if others don't have healthy boundaries, we can develop our own.

Integrity

Our lives will occasionally take center stage in family discussions or at the office, but usually they don't. Sometimes everybody's talkin' about me, but much more often they're not. What I mean is this: We exaggerate what people are thinking and saying about us. If people are talking about us a little, it's easy to think we're the only thing on their minds. (A little grandiose, don't you think?)

When we exaggerate the extent to which people are talking about us, we then may also exaggerate what they might be saying. We take a piece of what one person is saying and a piece of what another might have said, and soon we're trying to sort through a strange concoction of messages. If we have trouble turning down the volume on these voices, we're likely to feel quite confused.

If you struggle with low self-esteem or an unclear sense of identity, these amplified and exaggerated voices are going to cause you even more problems. If you haven't learned to quiet yourself and listen to your own voice and the voice of God, you stand an even greater risk of confusion.

We cannot look exclusively to others to help us sort out our thoughts. A few trusted friends may have a keen ability to help us listen to ourselves, but by and large, this is solitary work. We generally cannot look to others to help us develop a clear sense of identity. It doesn't work. We become even more fragmented in the process. We lose ourselves in the crowd.

Parker Palmer, whose writing I particularly appreciate, wrote a book titled *A Hidden Wholeness*. In it he writes poignantly about the issue of integrity: "When we understand integrity for what it is, we stop obsessing over moral codes of conduct and embark on the more demanding journey toward being whole." He makes special note of people who made difficult decisions and stood by them, such as Rosa Parks and Nelson Mandela. "You catch a glimpse of the beauty that arises when people refuse to live divided lives."[1]

One of our greatest powers is the power of choice. Every day we have the responsibility and privilege of making big and little decisions. Each decision we make is an exclamation point to the world of our existence. We each get to say...

"This is what I believe."

"This is what's important to me."

"This is what I hate."

"This is what I love."

"This is what I'd like from you."

"This is how you can help me."

These may seem like small decisions, but they are anything but that. Each choice, every announcement of what we believe, is one step closer to living with integrity, to being whole.

I have a choice to make regarding my boat. I can listen to 20 different voices and become confused by them. Or I can stop my persistent scrounging for advice, move in ways closer to the center of who I am, and live with the consequences of my choices.

Kelly has some choices facing her. She can listen to her family and let their discouragement turn her away from her courageous inclination, or she can hear their voices softly, knowing what they think but moving inexorably toward what will make her whole—living with integrity.

Never Defend or Debate

Your choices may be more challenging. They're not about boats or where to live. You worry about whether the church will approve of your choice to stop teaching a Sunday school class or what your friends and family might say about you leaving an abusive husband. You're pulled in different directions about whether to homeschool your children or send them to a Christian school or public school. You have questions about your faith.

If you're like me, you have a hunch about what is right for you, but you get bogged down when you listen to too many voices. You get befuddled when you believe everyone will talk about you disparagingly if you make the wrong choice.

Here's where we can get very confused. We know we want to do something, but we're pretty sure this action will meet with disapproval—and we can't stand that! So we mull over our choices again and again and again. Can you hear the wheels spinning in your brain? We invite criticism, creating even more inner chaos. We listen to the endless voices, challenging some and fighting off others.

I have an answer to this struggle—but it takes tremendous courage to follow this path. Here it is: *Never defend or debate with others about your choices.*

You may think, *Why shouldn't I defend my position? How can I possibly not explain myself to my friends and family? I need to stand up for what I think.*

Actually, if you defend yourself, you're in for worse trouble. I'll explain, thanking John Bradshaw for his brilliant insight into this issue in his book *Healing the Shame that Binds You*.

Bradshaw asserts that a very unhealthy situation occurs when we share our sacred kernel of truth with others and they, without invitation, criticize it. Let's again imagine Kelly sharing with her family that she's thinking of quitting her law practice and moving to California. Her family feels threatened and criticizes her decision, so they launch into a tirade about how she'll leave Mom alone, she'll never be able to start another law practice, and California will surely have another earthquake soon, ruining her whole plan. Kelly has to make a quick decision. She can...

- Soak up every word they say, letting their discouragement thwart her plans.

- Mull over their ideas, allowing them to make her feel crazy inside. What was she thinking, anyway?

- Listen to their advice and launch into a counterattack, defending her decision to move to California and hoping against hope they'll eventually agree with her.

- Listen in a detached manner, letting them know she hears their concerns but doesn't want to continue the conversation. She can let them know later what she decides.

What would you do if you were Kelly? How do you usually handle other people's opinions about your important decisions?

My first response has often been to listen to people's advice and then launch into a defensive counterattack, trying to make them see my point of view. I want them to agree with me, but that rarely works. I often end up feeling even more confused about my decision.

Bradshaw asserts that when you defend yourself, you let others make you feel ashamed. They want to criticize you, and if you start defending yourself, you'll take on some of that ridicule.

How do we not get lured into defending ourselves or debating with others? This is a tricky situation. I have a few ideas for you.

- Don't get into these situations in the first place. Become more adept at guarding your heart and sharing important information only with those you can count on to be careful with you. Learn to discern who is safe with your ideas and who isn't.

- Stop a conversation you see turning in a negative direction. If your friends and family begin offering unwanted advice, tell them you aren't seeking advice. Clarify that you are simply informing them about your possible actions.

- Listen to people and acknowledge their concerns without getting hooked into a long conversation. Tell them that you hear their concerns, and thank them for their input. But consciously reserve your own opinion. Carefully hold back, being very aware that you will walk away and decide what is best for you. Remind yourself that you know what is best for you, and others cannot possibly be in a position to tell you what to do.

Don't expect to learn these skills quickly. You might take years to perfect the art of expressing yourself without inviting or getting hooked by the opinions of others. To stop a conversation that is obviously turning against us takes great courage. Be kind to yourself as you grow in this area.

Public Embarrassment

What if people really *are* talking about you, and not in a kind way? How do you handle gossip or public criticism?

Most of us have been the topic of unkind table conversation at some time in our lives. However, as I mentioned at the start of this chapter, we tend to exaggerate how often and how negatively people are talking about us. We usually minimize the good things they say.

We all want to be liked. We want acceptance and approval. The key is to want acceptance but not need it so much that we allow it to dictate our behavior.

Not long ago I worked with a 30-year-old man, Gale, who was fired from his job for taking some tools off the job without permission. He hadn't really considered this stealing because he only wanted to borrow them for a home project. Nonetheless, his behavior was wrong. He knew it and readily admitted the wrongfulness of his actions.

Gale suffered extensively from this public humiliation. He lost a long-standing job that he enjoyed, and he was charged with theft.

"I hate being thought of as a thief," Gale told me early in our work together. "I'm not a thief," he said angrily. "That's just not who I am. I've given years of my life to this job, and I've never had a mark against me. Now the entire place is talking about me."

"What exactly do you mean by that?" I asked.

"I know those guys. I know how they think, and I know how they talk. I'm sure they think I'm a thief. They think I set out to rob the place and have been doing it for years. They're probably glad I got caught, and now they're laughing about me."

"Are you sure about that?" I asked inquisitively. "How do you know what they're thinking?"

"Well, I guess I don't know for sure, but I'd think that if someone else was charged with theft."

"Let's look closely at this, Gale," I said. "First, would you think of someone *only* as a thief? Or would you think that's just one part of his life?"

"When you put it that way, I guess I'd know he was more than just a thief."

"Exactly," I said. "Also, would you really label him a thief? Or might you wonder if this was a one-time event?"

"I don't know," Gale said. "I might think it was just a one-time thing, but I might wonder if he just got caught after doing it for years."

"My point too," I said. "We'd have lots of different thoughts running through our heads with lots of different possibilities."

"Yeah," he said.

"Finally," I continued, "would you really chide that person?"

"No, I suppose not," Gale said slowly. "I might wonder what prompted him to do it. I'd probably be glad he got caught. I might think of the mess it would make of his life."

"I bet other people can see your situation for what it is. You wrongfully took the tools home to use but had no thought of stealing them."

"I doubt others look at things that way," he persisted. "I'm sure everyone at the mill is running off at the mouth."

"Maybe so," I suggested. "But let me ask you another question. How long do you think they'll be talking about you?"

"A couple of months," he said. "Maybe more."

"Maybe less," I asserted. "Are you sure your situation is so important to people that they'll talk about you continuously for a couple of months?"

Gale began to loosen up in the chair.

"OK, maybe it just *seems* like people will be talking about me," he said.

"Exactly," I asserted. "We tend to amplify the problem in our minds and exaggerate our own importance. The truth of the matter is that we're pretty short-term news for folks. They've got other things to worry about than our problems."

With this I continued my line of thinking. "Do you sit home at night and talk about other people and their problems? Is that your typical dinner conversation?"

He hesitated as he considered the question. "Not really," he said a little embarrassed. "But we do talk about other people."

"For a week straight?"

"Probably not," he said. "I get your point."

Gale had to remind himself that he was not as important to the guys at the mill as he imagined. Gale and his challenges would be fleeting news and wouldn't last a week. Hardly for a day.

This is good news for us who worry about managing other people's opinions of us. We're just not as important to them as we think we might be.

Eleanor Roosevelt

Eleanor Roosevelt was born in New York City on October 11, 1884, the daughter of Anna Hall and Elliott Roosevelt, the younger brother of President Theodore Roosevelt. Eleanor was a shy and awkward child, starved for recognition and love. Her mother died when she was eight, and her father died when she was ten, so she was raised by her maternal grandmother.

Roosevelt attended a distinguished school for girls in England, where her self-confidence grew. After her return to the United States, her circle of friends included a distant cousin, Franklin Delano Roosevelt. They dated and eventually married in 1905, with her uncle, President Theodore Roosevelt, giving the bride away.

Having been raised in prominence, her marriage to Franklin Roosevelt catapulted her into the public spotlight. Her husband served in the New York Senate from 1910 to 1913, during which time she started her long career as political helpmate.

Eleanor Roosevelt could have chosen a more reserved life, but she learned about Washington and its ways while her husband served as assistant secretary of the Navy. When he was stricken with poliomyelitis in 1921, she tended him devotedly and became active in the state Democratic committee. From his successful campaign for governor in 1928 to the day of his death, she dedicated her life to his political interests and his well-being.

Eleanor Roosevelt quickly became one of the most revered women in American history. Many believe she transformed the role of first lady as she engaged in official entertaining, greeting thousands with charming friendliness. She broke precedent by holding press conferences, traveling with and without her husband, giving lectures, and even having her own radio show.

Naturally, all this activity made her a perfect target for criticism. Her political adversaries took shots at her, but her sincerity and grace endeared her to the public. As one of the first of the American presidents' wives to be outspoken, Eleanor Roosevelt took a lot of criticism for her behavior. Opinionated and vocal, she dared to say many things that were unpopular. If anyone had a right to be concerned about what others were saying, she did. Others *were* talking about her!

In spite of the rash of criticism she received, Roosevelt lived with integrity. She knew what she believed, and at a time when women were generally silent in public, she took a stand. She was a brave and daring woman who seemed to live her life fearlessly.

Detaching with Love

How did a socially awkward girl become a graceful, dignified, powerful woman in such a male-dominated culture? Didn't Roosevelt care what people thought of her? I suspect she cared, but she achieved a wonderful balance between caring and not caring too much. That is the goal for each of us: to appreciate acceptance without sacrificing our integrity for it. Roosevelt understood her purpose, and this strengthened her to pursue her passion in spite of the criticism she received.

"No one can make you feel inferior without your consent," she wrote in 1937.

Those words have caused me to pause and reflect on many occasions. You mean *no one* can demean us without us first granting them permission? Yes, this is the truth. We can achieve a place of inner stability and resolve where we care about others' opinions but don't live to attain their approval. As we see with Roosevelt, this is an enviable state.

This delicate balance is nearly impossible to achieve. We are insecure and inclined to make too much of others' opinions, so we make compromises we should not make. We take criticism too personally. We bend and shape our lives to fit public opinion. We bind our creativity in order to fit in. Consequently, we relinquish the possibility of greatness and diminish our integrity.

The apostle Peter struggled the same way we do. Desperate for approval, Peter had been Jesus' disciple for more than three years when he failed his first major test. During the grueling hours prior to Jesus' death, when Jesus needed a friend, Peter denied that he ever knew his

Master. Peter acted codependently, seeking other people's approval in spite of his own convictions.

Experiencing disgrace, Peter was given an opportunity to redeem himself, which he did. As time passes, Peter changes and grows from being temperamental and unsure of himself to becoming a rock in the church's foundation. His character strengthens and his courage firms. He stands up to the Pharisees and others who criticize him.

In one telling passage, we read about Peter healing a lame man, to the chagrin of the religious leaders. Peter, sure of himself and his convictions, lets the religious leaders have it: "Men of Israel, why does this surprise you? Why do you stare at us as if by our own power or godliness we had made this man walk? The God of Abraham, Isaac and Jacob, the God of our fathers, has glorified his servant Jesus" (Acts 3:12-13). Peter continues with an incredibly brave tongue-lashing that landed him in jail. Timid, frightened Peter had found a new strength— the power of the Holy Spirit had changed him.

Did Peter no longer care about others' opinions? Certainly not in the same way he had before. No longer did he live for acceptance and approval. As he led the formation of the church, he was now willing to have people talk about him. Did he ever struggle with this again? Yes—read his encounter with other Jewish Christians in Galatians 2:11-13.

Who's talking about you? What are they saying? My hope is that like Peter, you can learn to live without other people's admiration or approval.

We've explored the temptation to make too much of other people's impressions, and we've discovered the importance of being true to ourselves and our calling. In the next chapter we'll look at our tendency to believe our problems are bigger than others' and find out what we can do about it.

7

Emotional Myopia

What can we gain by sailing to the moon if we are not able to cross the abyss that separates us from ourselves? This is the most important of all voyages of discovery, and without it, all the rest are not only useless, but disastrous.

THOMAS MERTON

I am livid.

Walking out to my car this morning, I discovered a hotel advertising sign leaning against my car, with gashes evident where the sign had hit my car. After removing the sandwich board, I went in to inform hotel personnel and ask them to document the damage.

The hotel clerk was very friendly and empathetic. "I completely understand your frustration," she said, showing concern. "You've got a nice car. I'd hate it if something like this happened to me."

I felt immediate relief. She reassured me that the hotel would make things right.

A few minutes later I received a call from the front desk to my room. "I'm sorry, sir," she said slowly, "but the hotel manager says there is a sign out front saying 'Park at your own risk.' So we can't be held responsible for the damage to your car."

"What!" I said in disbelief. "I didn't see any sign like that. I'll be right down."

Grumbling to Christie as I left our room, I felt the blood rise in me. I marched down to the front desk and asked for clarification. I was directed to a small, barely noticeable sign 30 feet away from my car. I protested that they couldn't possibly expect any customer to see the sign, and even if they could, another sign of theirs had caused damage to my car. They were unwavering, and I bristled.

I walked out again to see this sign. Angry and frustrated, I wondered, *Were they in the right? Had I been in the wrong?* There was the sign in very small print and far enough away from where I parked that I could never have seen it. Another sign of theirs blew into my car, causing the damage. Still, they pointed fingers at me!

At this moment I'm waiting to talk to the management of the hotel firm, feeling very discouraged. The hotel is not likely to repair my car, so I can engage in a verbal battle, live with the damage, or pay a costly repair bill. All three options feel undesirable. I feel angry, frustrated, and vengeful. This incident has ruined my morning—a downer in the middle of a surprise weekend away arranged by my wife. I'm struggling with emotional myopia.

We all occasionally struggle with emotional myopia. An isolated event consumes our thoughts and stirs up unwanted emotions. Our objectivity is challenged, and our feelings take on a life of their own. We feel out of control.

Myopia is an optical condition of nearsightedness. Items that are close look clear, but things in the distance are blurry. This occurs when images are focused on the front of the retina rather than on the retina itself.

Emotional myopia occurs when we become fixated on our problems. We lack discernment and perspective, so our troubles seem more serious than they actually are. This is a common malady because we easily get caught up in our own pain. When we are distraught over some situation in our life, we couldn't care less about what is happening in the rest of the world, what is occurring across town, or even what is happening with our friends or family. We are only interested in reducing our pain.

As I mentioned in chapter 3, Christie and I recently got into a fight.

We rarely argue, but this was quite an exception. We not only had words, as you might recall, but also didn't speak to one another for several hours. I even left our home in an attempt to calm my frayed nerves.

During this time I lost touch with reality. That's not to say I went crazy; I just lost perspective. I couldn't think about anything but our fight. For a relatively short time, my emotions were overcome with pain, anger, frustration, and resentment. Just as when the hotel personnel made excuses for the scratches on my car, I was shortsighted. I had emotional myopia. In the midst of my anger—which often fuels emotional myopia—I had thoughts like these:

> *This isn't fair.*
>
> *I'm getting a bad rap.*
>
> *It's not my fault.*
>
> *I'm really angry with Christie.*
>
> *Others don't struggle with their marriages like we're struggling.*

I had a sense that my thoughts were distorted, but during those few hours our problems seemed much bigger than they were.

Fortunately, Christie and I are able to make up fairly quickly. In a very short time I went from feeling as if we were doomed to remembering the good things about our marriage. I went from myopic to having a clear vision. I went from believing that no one else struggles the way we do to realizing that our experience is normal. I was able to see that this was not a catastrophe.

A Mood

Moods fuel emotional myopia. Moods have been called temporary insanity because during our bad moods we rehearse bad feelings, think negative thoughts, turn manageable problems into catastrophes, and generally lose perspective.

Bad moods can make us feel crazy. Bad moods can make us forget the love we feel for our mate, wonder why we live in the house we do, complain about our work, and even question our sanity. We're ready to label ourselves bipolar because of our seesawing emotions.

Can you relate? Do you ever lose perspective? Do your problems ever seem much bigger than anyone else's you know? Do you ever question your sanity? A bad mood can do all of that to us.

Let's look at a typical situation of emotional myopia.

Jared is a 25-year-old man who is engaged to Lisa, a wonderful young woman from our church. I've known them both for more than a year. I've watched them in several settings as they showed obvious affection for each other, joked around, and seemed very compatible. I assumed things were going well for them until the pastor called and asked if I'd see them.

"What's up?" I asked the pastor.

"I'm not sure," the pastor said. "I think Jared may have cold feet. He's thinking about calling off their engagement, and I think he'd appreciate being able to talk about it."

"I'd be happy to," I told my pastor. A short time later I saw Jared in my office.

Although casually dressed in loose-fitting jeans and wearing a ball cap, Jared appeared unsettled as he looked at the pictures in my waiting room.

"Come on in," I said to Jared. "Good to see you."

"Yeah, I guess," Jared offered cautiously.

As he came into my office, he took a moment to look around, paying special attention to my framed degrees.

"You spent some time in school," Jared said, looking at me for my response.

"Yep—I'm glad it's behind me."

"Do you specialize in a particular area?" he asked.

"I like to work with relationships a lot. I like to help couples work out problems. That's probably the counseling I like the best."

"You write books too," he added.

"Yes, I like to write," I said. "So what about you? You didn't come here to talk about me."

"Pastor Paul sent me here," Jared said slowly, still looking around the room but seeming more relaxed. "I guess I'm here because I'm confused about Lisa. Things are kind of out of control."

"You and Lisa are having problems?" I asked.

"Yes and no. Sometimes we are and other times we're not. Sometimes I think our problems are normal, but at other times I can hardly think straight. Every now and then I just want to bag the whole relationship. I need to figure out what to do."

"I'm glad you're here, Jared," I said. "I can help you sort out your problems with Lisa. We'll figure out when and why you feel confused, and that will help you make good decisions about what to do."

"That would be great," Jared said. "Sometimes our problems seem huge to me. They're all I can think about. If we've had a fight, I can't focus on my work the next day. I get carried away and start thinking the worst."

I smiled as Jared shared his feelings. "You're not alone, Jared. I can assure you that everybody has their issues." I paused for a moment to let my words sink in. "And when it comes to relationships, it's a wonder to me that anyone gets along for more than fifteen minutes. We're created so differently. How long have you and Lisa been going together?"

"A little over a year. The first six months were incredible, and then we started having issues. One thing after another, with nothing really getting settled. When I think about our problems, I get bummed out. But when I think of the good times, I want to be with her forever. It's like I'm on a roller coaster."

"I can relate," I told Jared. "Like I said, relationships are tough work. But just because you guys are struggling doesn't mean you're not right for each other. It probably means you have issues that need to be resolved, and you also need to learn to keep things in perspective. You might be having problems, but problems can be solved."

"I don't know," Jared began. "We're not solving our problems, and it's killing us. I've always tended to get a little moody. Lisa gets moody too, and when we're moody together, watch out."

"What happens then?" I asked.

"We go into a free fall," Jared explained. "She says things about me, I get upset, I say things about her, she gets upset, and pretty soon we're questioning whether we're right for each other. We both slip into a bad mood pretty easy, and we don't even think about the good times."

Jared and I spent the next few sessions talking about bad moods. We discussed the way moods can be like temporary insanity as we lose perspective. Moods cause us to see the world in a distorted way, often amplifying our problems and minimizing our ability to manage them. We saw that moods are not an accurate representation of reality.

After several weeks of meeting together, Jared began to regain his emotional footing. We decided to invite Lisa to join us. Together we discovered they had a very solid relationship and still shared a love and commitment for each other. They began to learn skills to stop the slide when things became overly emotional. They started learning how to keep things in perspective when they were angry, discouraged, or frustrated with one another.

The Emotional Slide

Emotions become very unruly at times. In fact, they often seem to have a life of their own. As I've written in *The Power of Emotional Decision Making,* emotions are "energy in motion." Feelings have their own energy.

This is both good news and bad news. We enjoy riding the wave of pleasant emotions, but we would rather avoid wiping out in a swell of painful ones.

Jared, for example, was caught in a swirl of discouragement. As his energy in motion picked up steam, he slid into a negative mood. Feeling confused by his discouragement—and as we've seen, we can be confused by our feelings—he felt worse and worse. He was unable to put his feelings and thoughts in perspective, so he began questioning his relationship with Lisa.

We can all relate with Jared. We've been caught in the vortex of powerful emotions and felt carried away by them. These unruly emotions take on a life of their own.

Many biblical characters rode an emotional roller coaster. Elijah crashed and burned after running from the angry Queen Jezebel. Exhausted and discouraged, he slipped into a situational depression, asking God to take his life. Talk about emotional myopia. As soon as he rested and had a bite to eat, the world looked much better.

How about David, hiding in caves as he ran from King Saul? Certainly he slipped into feeling dejected, wondering if God had forsaken him. He needed rest and encouragement to regain perspective.

Times of moodiness, when our emotions run amok, can make us wonder if we're going crazy. We feel vulnerable, at the mercy of these "horrible, terrible, no good, very bad" emotions.

Split Personality

Our unruly moods and negative emotions make us feel fragile. We feel out of control and frustrated by our unmanageable feelings. We don't want to feel discouraged. We don't want to be swept off our feet by an angry mood. We don't want to pout and feel resentful. We don't want to cry!

To make matters worse, we wrestle not only with individual feelings but also with a larger mood—often a composite of many different emotions. On top of our original feelings about a specific situation, we feel overtaken by a mood that brings feelings of guilt, exasperation, and confusion.

Who is this person with these feelings, we wonder? Up one minute and down the next. We really must be disturbed, we surmise. We must have something biochemically wrong with us. What kind of foul mood is this? Why can't we shake these feelings and get on with life? We feel as if we're losing our grip on reality. These moods can be very disconcerting.

Barbara De Angelis, in her book *How Did I Get Here?* explains that we must continually be learning how to think about ourselves.

> What is there for us to do during our time on earth that is more crucial to our sense of inner peace and more central to our experience of wholeness than knowing and understanding ourselves?...In spite of our hope that once we figure out who and what we are, we can relax and cruise through the rest of our journey, it just doesn't happen this way. Instead, we change. Circumstances change. Other people change, and all of these changes change us even more.[1]

De Angelis is saying that we're all on a journey to understand ourselves. Actually, I think we're on a journey to understand our selves—our different parts. We're all on a journey to make sense of our disparate feelings and annoying moods.

So you don't have a split personality even though you don't understand these moods and slippery feelings. You're not going crazy in spite of the fact that you can't harness those unruly emotions at times. Those emotions are natural aspects of your personhood and have a life of their own.

I should make something clear. I agree with De Angelis that on our quest to know ourselves, we will never be able to hit the cruise control. But we can become increasingly familiar with our emotions and thoughts so that we're less likely to be ambushed by them. We can achieve a certain amount of mastery over our emotions and thoughts, and this can ease the effect of challenging moods.

The apostle Paul, whose letters reveal that he had his share of moods and frustrations, learned to "take captive every thought to make it obedient to Christ" (2 Corinthians 10:5). We can be encouraged that as we are filled by the Spirit of God and transformed by the renewing of our minds, we can learn to manage our emotions. The fruit of the Spirit brings stability to our personality.

Emotional Crises

The quest to know and understand ourselves becomes all the more baffling in the middle of crises. These are times when we really do feel out of control—and yet we're really not as crazy as we think. We need not expect that we will always react calmly in the middle of a personal loss, transition, or catastrophic illness.

My work as a clinical psychologist includes helping people cope with crises. Nearly every day, I walk alongside someone who is suffering from a broken relationship, divorce, marital or family conflict, or even death. We may daydream about sailing through situations like these with ease, but we cannot expect to act like machines.

Recently I worked with a 35-year-old woman who was abjectly distraught over the possibility of losing her seven-year marriage. Kendra, a thin, anxious woman, appeared tired and worn when I first saw her. She wasted no time telling me why she had made an appointment.

"You've got to help me save my marriage," she said, her speech pressured and her eyes wide with anxiety. "My husband says he doesn't want to work on our marriage. I know I can fix the things he's complaining about. I know I haven't been the wife he needs, but I can be. He said he'd come in once, and you have to make things work."

"Slow down a little, Kendra," I said, trying to comfort her. "I can see this is really upsetting you. I need to hear more about your marriage and what has happened."

Kendra told me about her marriage and her five-year-old son named Jacob. She explained that she and her husband had been verbally aggressive with one another and had exhibited patterns of unfaithfulness.

"I know I can be mean and spiteful in our fighting," Kendra said. "I know that's the main reason he left. But I can change. I've got to change."

Kendra began sobbing. Slumping into a near-fetal position in one of my chairs, Kendra was aching. She wanted her husband back desperately, yet their situation sounded dismal. With thoughts and emotions spinning out of control, Kendra was sleeping poorly, losing weight, and missing work. She hoped I could perform some magic in their marriage.

Of course, no quick-and-easy answers will solve Kendra's problem. Her husband left after years of turmoil. Theirs wasn't a minor hurdle to hop over; it was a mountain that they would have to scale. She would need to find ways to soothe her troubled spirit while painstakingly exploring possibilities for reconciliation with her husband.

In the meantime, Kendra had to determine how to manage the emotional myopia this crisis had caused. How would she settle the tempest that raged inside her while she traversed a difficult crossing in her marriage? Let's consider a few of the ways we can find peace when our world is temporarily in chaos.

1. We all need internal anchors. When things outside are unstable, we need something to keep us from being blown away in the storm. As surely as a boat needs an anchor for stable mooring in the winds and waves, we need anchors for our soul. Take some time to consider who and what might sustain you in unstable times.

2. We all need support. None of us can make it alone. We need friends and family we can lean on when the going gets rough. We need people we can call on, sometimes in the middle of the night, when we simply can't shut our brain down. Do you have friends and family like that?

3. We all need faith. Specifically, we need faith in a God who promises to see us through to the other side of the storm. Just as surely as God was a refuge to Moses and was his shelter in "the cleft of the rock," we need to know that God is personal, close, and willing to give us wisdom for our difficult times.

4. We need to trust that our raging feelings and thoughts will settle. We want to feel better *now*, but you have probably experienced enough of life to know that this too shall pass. You can listen to your thoughts and feelings and use them to bring clarity, but you cannot make your feelings settle in an instant. You cannot clear your thoughts with one sentence. You can, however, trust that your thoughts and feelings will eventually calm.

5. We need self-soothing skills. You may settle your nerves with a hot bath or a cool walk. Compile a list of things that help you feel better. Perhaps you can call a friend or write in your journal. Maybe you prefer to pray through the psalms. Find out what brings relief for you when emotions spin out of control.

6. We need to know that God can use this situation for our good. Yes, whatever is happening, regardless of how uncomfortable, it can benefit us. "In all things God works for the good of those who love him, who have been called according to his purpose" (Romans 8:28). How comforting to know that these roller-coaster emotions, this challenging situation, or this incredible loss can be used for our benefit and for God's glory.

Kendra left my office with tear-stained eyes. She wanted a shortcut through her crisis. She wanted quick relief. She wanted to avoid what Scott Peck calls "legitimate suffering." But I knew that easy answers wouldn't be honest answers. She needed to stay in the crucible if she was going to learn anything that might help her with her husband or her future. I couldn't give her the promise she desperately wanted.

Emotional Distortions

Even in the best of times, we can easily misinterpret information. Our ability to distort information in the worst of times is even higher, making us feel crazy.

Our intricate brains can process and analyze billions of pieces of data in seconds, but they can also jumble that information into an unrecognizable mass. As if we had dumped the pieces of a jigsaw puzzle onto the floor, we review our messy lives and wonder what on earth we were thinking.

Add a healthy dose of emotion to a situation, and soon we're left to puzzle over what we are experiencing. One moment we think this, and a few seconds later we think that. Having two diverging thoughts can be maddening enough, but what if we have multiple thoughts and layers of emotions at the same time? It's enough to make us feel crazy.

But we're not crazy. We've been wired to process countless divergent thoughts, numerous disagreeable feelings, and even some random experiences as well. We are capable of incredible acts of creative thinking, but we can also make quite a mess of things. We can listen to someone speak and then distort the information into almost unrecognizable form. We can repeat back what someone has just said, word for word, and still distort the speaker's meaning. We can listen to and understand someone and then "remember" that information in a completely different way than the speaker presented it. We twist and contort the message, often causing division and significant conflict.

In short, the possibility for emotional distortion is endless. Let's consider some of the ways we jumble our thoughts and feelings, creating feelings of craziness.

Emotional Flooding

Sometimes we are too close to our feelings, or our feelings are simply too intense for us to manage effectively. This often occurs during a crisis.

I met with a young man today for an emergency session. Jerry, a hard-working Sheetrock installer, burly and strong, looked tired and worn. He nearly insisted on being hospitalized because of the anxiety he has felt since an intense encounter with his wife last night.

Jerry was in a horrible mood, feeling dejected after his wife confronted him. He admitted that he had acquired thousands of dollars in gambling debts from his addiction to pull tabs, and his wife had found his credit card bill. Furious, she told him to pack his clothes immediately and move out.

Jerry was experiencing an emotional crisis, to be sure, as undoubtedly was his wife. Both were reacting emotionally to their particular crises. Jerry faced an imminent separation from his wife and two young children as well as a mountain of guilt from the emotional and financial costs of his addiction. His wife faced an uncertain financial future as well as fears from their likely separation.

As I met with Jerry, I encouraged him with the truth that this too shall pass. His wife was clearly furious with him and wanted him out of her sight, but her feelings would calm, and that could lead her to make a more rational decision. He too needed to adjust to being separated so that he and his wife could talk over their future.

This crisis caused emotional distortions for both Jerry and his wife. What they felt today is different from what they will feel tomorrow. I encouraged Jerry not to make any rash decisions and to move slowly. We hope his wife will do the same.

Losing Control

Emotional flooding leads to feelings of losing control, and this is a horrible feeling. No one wants to feel his or her life unraveling. Whether we have anticipated a crisis, or something entirely unpredicted happens to disrupt our world, the loss of normalcy creates inner chaos.

Too often, we overreact in times of crisis. Instead of *feeling* our feelings, allowing them their expression, we try to control them. This almost always creates even more problems. Melody Beattie describes a more helpful approach in her book *Finding Your Way Home:*

> We don't want our feelings to control us. But they do, until we feel them. It doesn't mean we need to run around dramatically displaying every emotional current that passes through us, although that's a good way to get in touch and help the emotional release. Feeling our feelings means we bow to them. We acknowledge them.[2]

This takes practice. In the moment, especially if we're not used to strong emotions, we can feel quite confused by feelings we haven't felt in a long time. With time and experience, however, we can befriend these feelings, honor them, and see what they have to teach us. As we do this, we actually regain control of our lives.

Pathologizing Our Feelings

We also experience emotional distortion when we believe something is wrong with us because we feel the way we do. We tell ourselves we shouldn't feel what we're feeling. The result is that we not only feel overwhelmed but also feel guilty. In addition to feeling frightened, confused, and slightly panicked, we are ashamed for those feelings. Can you see the irony in this?

In truth, we need not feel guilty for *any* emotion. Emotions aren't right or wrong, although actions can be. Assuming you don't act on every single emotion you feel, you need not feel guilty for having the feelings you do.

As Beattie says, try bowing to your feelings. Try asking them what they want to tell you. Prepare a soft place for your feelings to rest, and see if they begin to ease and perhaps even dissipate. As I've said, a feeling denied is intensified. One sure way to feel even crazier is to attempt to suppress your feelings or to tell yourself that you shouldn't be feeling what you're feeling. Instead of taking these destructive actions, tell yourself that your feelings make sense. Others would feel the same way if they were in your shoes.

No One Understands Me

Another emotional distortion is to tell yourself that no one understands what you're experiencing. Telling yourself that you're utterly unique will make you feel strange, peculiar, and yes, a little bit crazy.

The truth is, your experiences are a lot like other people's, and those who endure circumstances similar to yours are likely to feel the way you do. If you don't understand that, you will feel odd and therefore a tad crazy. You feel crazier when you rehearse the notion that no one could possibly understand what you are going through. Telling yourself that you are different will make you feel different.

I've discovered in more than 30 years of counseling that we're remarkably similar to one another. We have remarkably similar experiences with remarkably similar reactions. This is what makes support groups so powerful. I recommend them for nearly everyone I see in counseling. I recommended a Gamblers Anonymous group for Jerry, an eating disorders support group for an obese woman trying to manage her weight, and an Alcoholics Anonymous group for a man trying to maintain his sobriety and for his wife, who felt crazy trying to understand her husband's addiction. Support groups remind us that we're quite normal in our reactions, and they help us out of our emotional myopia.

I Must Be Losing My Mind

A sudden surge of emotion, combined with a lack of support, can lead to emotional myopia and the fear of losing our minds. A blast of emotion almost always leads to instability.

I am a novice sailor. A fine line separates the feeling of exhilaration that comes with tacking away from the wind as the boat heels close to the water, and the fear that I might capsize at any moment. Experience with emotion leads to confidence, but even an experienced sailor occasionally has to pull back, tacking closer to the wind and stabilizing the boat. We must do the same thing at times with our emotions.

In times of crisis, when emotions feel unruly and unmanageable, we may feel as if we're losing our minds, but we're not. Emotions have never made anyone crazy. This truth can be a powerful antidote to the fear of becoming mentally unstable. Imagine reassuring yourself with these thoughts in the midst of emotional turmoil:

- *This feeling is normal in this situation.*
- *Others would likely feel the same way in a similar situation.*
- *These feelings can help me make good decisions.*
- *I can manage these feelings and even soothe myself in the midst of them.*

We must remind ourselves that these feelings are part of our healing process, regardless of how unmanageable they feel.

William Bridges, author of the book *Transitions,* shares about the almost unbearable turmoil he experienced during his wife's illness and eventual death. Bridges couldn't eat, sleep, or process his emotions effectively. He was overwhelmed with grief, and his life became disorganized. He felt crazy. In time, however, he began to reorganize his life—a life without his beloved wife.

During times of transition we do better if we *expect* our emotions to be unruly. We should expect to have fuzzy thinking, racing thoughts, and sluggish energy. We must give our emotions a place to exist without harsh judgment, to express themselves in a natural way. We must remind ourselves that we're not losing our minds.

Things Will Never Be OK

If yesterday was painful and today isn't any better, we naturally project these thoughts and feelings into the future. We tell ourselves things will never be OK. This is what Jerry told himself when his wife asked him to leave. It is what many of us tell ourselves when the outlook appears bleak.

The older I get, the more I value my parents' platitude, "You'll feel better in the morning. This crisis will pass, and you'll come out the other side stronger than ever."

These words were particularly soothing during a difficult time in my life. When I was working on my doctorate, my teenage sons were demanding, and life seemed to be crashing in around me, I couldn't see around the next corner. I could only see yesterday and today, and they appeared dismal. But my parents, with years of wisdom and experience, reminded me of several truths. I grabbed onto these for dear life:

- This crisis will pass.
- My parents love me and are available to support me.
- God will never leave me or forsake me.

- God will be a source of wisdom and strength in the days ahead.

- Joy will return to my life.

These truths are hard to hear with emotional myopia. When all we can see is what is right in front of our noses, we are likely to feel discouraged. Understanding our shortsightedness brings us hope. We can embrace the promises of God and the truth that our crisis will pass.

My crisis passed. I endured with much prayer, support, and wisdom from God. I reached the other side of the chasm and am stronger and happier today. The same can be true for you.

Remembering

One of the most powerful antidotes to emotional myopia and feelings of craziness is to remember where we have been and where we are going.

Whenever I am driving and get lost, I pull to the side of the road and take out my trusty map. I reorient myself. Where am I? Where have I been, and where do I want to go? Once I am reoriented, I jump back onto the highway and head for my destination.

Emotional myopia plays havoc with our sense of direction. Emotional flooding causes us to make impulsive moves that exacerbate our problems. Sinking into a pit of discouragement or a bad mood makes me lose my momentum and sense of direction. At those times I must calm myself down, settle my jangled nerves, and remember where I am and where I'm going.

We often forget the many blessings occurring in our lives. We forget that we are on a safe path or that we have the skills to create safety in our lives. Too often we feel that our lives are out of control and that we're passengers on a treacherous journey.

Remember the story of the disciples being caught in a storm on the Sea of Galilee? They had pushed away from the crowds, and Jesus had fallen asleep in the bow of the boat. Suddenly a squall came up, and the waves whipped the boat furiously. The disciples were understandably frightened.

They awakened Jesus, who appeared to be indignant at having been awakened from His nap. After rebuking the wind and waves, which immediately calmed, He confronts the disciples. "Why are you so afraid? Do you still have no faith?" (Mark 4:40).

This story contains a powerful lesson. Jesus asks the disciples to *remember.* Remember who is the Master of the wind and waves. Remember who has guided them to safety dozens of times before. Remember who has promised never to leave them helpless. Remember.

Emotional myopia causes us to forget. We pay attention to the flooded feeling we have instead of the harbor on the horizon. We forget that we have friends and family for support and that God is just a whisper away.

Regaining Emotional Stability

When the winds and waves are too much for my small sailboat, I pull down the sails, batten the hatches, and head for safe harbor. That is what we must do when the storms in our lives make us feel crazy. Let's consider a few practical steps for loosening the grip of emotional myopia.

1. Get support. Yes, this is advice I give for nearly any problem. Holding hands with friends and family always lessens the craziness of a crisis. Sharing feelings with those who truly understand helps dilute the power of the emotion.

2. Get out of the storm. Whatever is causing the distress and emotional flooding must be stopped. Get away from work for a few days. Stop talking with your mate about the heated issue. Exercise and find creative ways to take a break from the trouble you find yourself in.

3. Try to see the bigger picture. Narrow views reinforce emotional myopia. Seek outside counsel to help you see beyond the current situation. Listen to a few trusted people's points of view on your situation. Work at expanding your perspective.

4. Rest. A good night's sleep can do wonders to help clear your mind. Sometimes we must stop working on a problem. We need a plutonium box into which we place the cares of the day, leaving them until we can return to them refreshed and ready to tackle them with a renewed mind. We need to trust our Master, who is fully capable of managing our winds and waves.

You've got problems. I've got problems. Your problems are unique to you, and mine are unique to me. Yours are no more serious than mine, and mine are no more serious than yours. Our task is to lessen our emotional myopia and keep things in perspective. You've learned how to do that in this chapter.

In the next chapter we'll talk about the problem of secrets, how they can make us feel crazy, and what to do about them.

8

If You
Only Knew

*When it's over, I want to say: all my life
I was a bride married to amazement.
I was a bridegroom taking the world into my arms.*

Mary Oliver

Standing in the security line at the airport, a woman turned around and abruptly asked, "What are you staring at?"

Caught off guard, I didn't realize I had been watching her.

"Nothing," I said quickly, turning away.

The woman had caught my attention. Her hair was tucked neatly in a bun, her skin was tanned and wrinkled, and she walked stooped over. Fragile and worn, she appeared to be a hundred and two years old. She was dressed sharply in a dark red suit, bracelets dangling from both wrists.

Her age wasn't what attracted my attention, however. It was her attitude.

Acting like the Queen for a Day, she ordered her equally frail husband around, snapped at the security personnel for asking to inspect her luggage, and scowled impatiently at the people ahead of her in line. I must have been staring at her when she barked at me.

Several minutes later I thought of many things I would have enjoyed saying to her, but it was too late. She was walking down the concourse as briskly as she could with her husband in tow.

I don't know the woman, but I've made up a story about her.

Virginia Clements Stone has a lot of money—old money! She lives in an established area of Chicago in a several-million-dollar townhouse near the shores of Lake Michigan. Her husband, Willford, made a lot of money as a businessman, but most of her wealth came from an inheritance.

Virginia was raised in private schools, living a life of luxury. She's too old to play golf, but she still goes to the country club every day to play bridge and enjoy a drink or two or three. She has been treated like royalty since childhood and still demands privileges.

Her husband has long since lost his zest for life. Though he was quite a successful banker, his wife never misses an opportunity to remind him that the privileges they enjoy come from her inheritance, not his income. In times past he countered her barbs with sharp words of his own; in recent years he has all but given up trying to assert his opinion. Her years of nagging and scolding have made him miserable.

She drinks too much, but no one ever comments on it. They're too polite. She is a philanthropist and tells everyone about the money she gives to her church and various charities. She is a Christian, but she is blind to her own faults and quick to see the faults of others.

Virginia felt a twinge of embarrassment when I noticed the way she treated people. She has a Christian image to maintain and can't tolerate the thought that anyone would think she is mean-spirited and vengeful. She is clearly self-righteous.

Beneath the surface, Virginia is angry and painfully sad, though she will never admit to it. Her two children, also raised with privilege, have turned against her. Her son and daughter, both well-educated, rarely visit or call. They have tired of her tyranny and the way she controls their father. She is furious that they secretly call him. She believes her husband, Willford, has pitted their children against her. She never lets on to her friends at the club and church that she is depressed.

You may think I've woven together an impossibly eccentric personality. Virginia even sounds a bit theatrical to me. But as they say, the truth is stranger than fiction. My story is contrived, but the story line comes from people I have counseled. I have no idea how this woman lives or if any of my imaginings are true, but there are plenty of people whose lives mimic my story about Willford and Virginia.

Sick as Our Secrets

In the story I've constructed, we are naturally critical of Virginia Clements Stone. She is an unlikeable person. But then again, we don't know the whole story. Why would this woman act so mean? Why would her husband allow such disrespectful behavior? We can only speculate, and chances are we'd be at least partially wrong.

What is true, however, is that we've all got skeletons in the closet. We all hide some aspects of our character and some episodes from our past. We're only as sick as our secrets, but our secrets keep us sick.

I've discovered through my work as a psychologist that the most righteous are not nearly as righteous as they appear, and the darkest individuals have redeeming qualities. The world is only black and white in our imagination. Someone has said that if we truly knew each other, our criticisms would fall away. We would realize we are not all that different, and we're not as crazy as we think.

My posturing began early in life. I was always the kind of kid who did a little of everything but excelled at very little. I played sports, but I was too short to play competitive basketball, too skinny to be formidable in football, and not strong enough to hit a baseball with any force.

My mediocrity extended to academics. I was smart enough to get by but certainly no intellectual standout. I could learn nearly anything, but most of the time I was clumped squarely in the middle of the pack.

But I seemed gifted in one area. My parents often told me that I could charm the socks off anyone. I realized I had "personality" and used every ounce of it to my advantage.

This may sound like an enviable trait, and it certainly can be, but personality can also be used for manipulation, and I've done more than my share of manipulating throughout my life. This was a secret aspect of my character that I didn't want to reveal or explore. I'd much rather hear people say, "What a charming guy," than "He certainly is manipulative."

My secret life of emotional manipulation picked up steam when I started working on my doctorate. Smart enough to compete academically, I found ways to use my charm to my full advantage. With tunnel vision, I rationalized that I had to work long hours because I was raising a family and wanted them to have the finer things in life. The truth of the matter was that I was addicted to work, accumulations, and success. I used my personality to manipulate people into feeling sorry for me. But the manipulation backfired. The more people felt sorry for me, the more I worked.

From the outside I looked exactly like I wanted to look—educated, successful, and prosperous. But on the inside, where no one could see, I was trying to silence old messages I believed: I had to be more, do more, and prove myself. No one had any idea I was fighting these inner demons. All they could see was a man with a Stephen Covey planner, a copy of *Dress for Success,* and a tireless attitude.

I had a house in the country, two delightful boys, and a marriage that looked good, so no one imagined my house of cards would one day collapse. In 1990 I became fatigued and unable to continue working at my previous pace. My addiction had caught up to me with considerable cost to my family life, my health, and my self-respect.

For years I kept my emotional collapse a secret. How could I, a well-known psychologist, admit to struggling with work addiction? How could I openly share that I participated in a men's 12-step group? Shouldn't I have been able to heal myself? Alone with my shame, I felt isolated, sick, and lonely. I couldn't let others know that my life was not working. I didn't want to appear weak, ineffective, or unable to solve my own problems. I had more than a bit of pride.

In my men's group, which I attended weekly for seven years, I learned that we're only as sick as our secrets. I learned that other men struggle with work addiction, posturing, and trying to look good. I learned that they were a lot like me. I wasn't as crazy as I thought, and I didn't have to keep my secret anymore.

Hiding

I now see that my life had been spiraling out of control for years. My work slowly invaded every aspect of my life, insidiously eroding my boundaries, my health, and my psyche. But I effectively hid this from others, or so I thought.

My hiding wasn't nearly as effective as I believed. It never is. Adam and Eve couldn't hide from an omnipresent God after their debacle. Virginia Clements Stone hoped in vain that no one would see her anger, abusive control, and tremendous sadness. And my own sins were more obvious to others than to me. My weaknesses and failures slowly became obvious to those concerned enough to notice. I tried to hide from the scrutiny of others, thinking they weren't seeing what was obvious. But they saw because David Hawkins' life was out of control.

As much as we try to hide the truth from others, we really can't do it for long. We may believe we're presenting a certain image, but anyone who is around us for long can see through our facade.

Sadly, all of our hiding, dodging, and posturing increase our feelings of craziness. We become less and less sure of ourselves. The more images we try to portray to others, the more confused we become about our true identity.

Several years ago I was a member of a church caught up in image. From the leadership down to the congregation, everyone lived the prosperity gospel. The pastor preached that if you were righteous enough, God would bless you. If you looked the part, you were the part. Image was everything. I can't direct all or even most of the responsibility at the pastor, though he led the congregation. We were all anxious to hear how we could receive the blessings God supposedly promised to give us.

The pastor's message was simple, and I had seen televangelists use it when I was growing up: If I trusted in the Lord, remained obedient to Him and to the church's teachings, and had enough faith, I would be blessed beyond measure. You have undoubtedly heard lines like these before.

I was invited to be part of the inner circle of this church. The pastor trusted me as one of his friends. People warned me about his manipulation, but I was lured by the possibility of being blessed by God and of receiving this powerful and influential man's recognition.

Needless to say, I was soon disappointed. The closer I came to my pastor, the more I could see behind his posturing, and I realized he was building his own kingdom rather than cooperating with God, who was building a very different kingdom. I began to see the dangers and fallacies of his life more clearly. He was not a happy man, but had devoted himself to a greedy quest for power and control. He didn't seem to be pursuing righteousness and the appropriate leadership of his family and congregation. Other people's admiration was more important to him. I became disappointed and ultimately left the church.

I was soured and discouraged, but as time has passed, I've had other feelings. I can see that this man was really hiding from his own feelings of insecurity. I could see myself in his desperate pursuit of success. I could sense the craziness he must have felt, preaching one thing and living another.

I came to see that all of us are not that much different from each other. I'd like to believe I'm not at all like this manipulative man, but the truth is that I do have similarities. He disappointed me; I've disappointed others. He lacked sincerity; I've lacked sincerity. He lived a duplicitous life; I've lived a double life as well.

I also feel sorry for this man and his family. Hiding from others is no fun. To always be on stage and hope others don't see through the facade is exhausting. Continually trying to convince others to believe a lie isn't easy. Living with the sense of insecurity that comes from this incredible self-deception is painful.

Self-Deception

To feel crazy from leading a double life is one thing, but to deceive ourselves is quite another. When purposely leading a double life, at least we usually know we're hiding something from others.

What about the feelings of craziness resulting from self-deception? After all, I really believed my motives were pure when I was in the throes of my work addiction. I was making myself crazy, but I didn't know it at the time. How much of our behavior and actions stem from motives and feelings we aren't aware of?

Much of my critical thinking about my former pastor is based on the presumption that he had some sense of his double life. I assumed he knew he was packing around a heavy load by posturing and protecting his image. But what if he didn't have a clue about all of this? What if he really believed everything he was saying? What if he really thought he was "all that"?

We've seen that the prophet Jeremiah says some harsh words to us about this matter. "The heart is deceitful above all things and beyond cure. Who can understand it?" (Jeremiah 17:9). In other words, we will never comprehend some things about the inner workings of our heart, and those inner urges and strivings can make us feel kind of crazy.

Parker Palmer says that secret-keeping children become secret-keeping adults, running the risk of becoming "armored adults." Here is a partial list of the price we pay for such armor:

- We sense that something is missing in our lives but don't know what it is, so we search the world for something that fits.

- We feel fraudulent or even invisible because we don't know who we really are, but we know that the image we project isn't accurate.

- We project our inner darkness on others, turning them into enemies and making the world a more dangerous place.

- Our inauthenticity and projections make real relationships impossible, so we become lonely.

- Our contributions to the world—especially through the work we do—are tainted by duplicity and deprived of life-giving energies of the true self.[1]

Parker's book title says it all—*A Hidden Wholeness*. He suggests that the craziness we feel from our posturing, hiding, and self-deception is unnecessary. Wholeness is available to us all if we will honestly face these problems.

Shame

Why do we posture even though we end up paying such a heavy price? Why do we hide from everyone, when in fact most of what we're hiding will find its way to the light of day? "Be sure that your sin will find you out," the Scripture says (Numbers 32:23). We can run and hide for only so long.

We run and hide because, like Adam and Eve, we are ultimately naked and ashamed. Adam and Eve covered themselves because they felt ashamed for what they had done. When God confronted them, Adam blamed his actions on Eve, and Eve blamed the serpent.

Every time I read the Genesis account of the Fall and I reach the part where Adam and Eve have sinned and flee from God, I want to gently offer them counsel.

"Hey, Adam and Eve," I say kindly. "Stop running from God. He can see everything you've done, and He's willing to talk things over."

Their reply, of course, would be to offer resistance.

"No way," they say in unison. "He'll never understand what we've done. We've made a royal mess of things."

"Yeah, that's right," I'd say. "Your actions missed the mark. You got caught up in trying to be more than you are. But I'm pretty sure God understands and will accept you back into fellowship with Him."

"Naw," Adam says forcefully. "We're going to hide from Him and cover up with a good story if He does catch up to us."

"You're wasting your time, you guys," I'd say. "It's better to simply fess up, take responsibility, and get on with life."

But I can't be critical of Adam and Eve, because I've done everything they've done. My actions often miss the mark, and I go into hiding. I can't really say I would have acted any differently than they did.

We've been taught to feel so bad and so ashamed for our failings that we naturally suppress, deny, and make excuses for our faults. Instead of simply acknowledging them, making appropriate changes, and getting on with things, we cover one wrong with another and heap denial upon denial.

In fact, our society reinforces denial. We deny the pain we experience and choose from myriad escapes and addictions to soothe our agony. We're all suffering and struggling with shame with few legitimate ways to heal.

The more we try to escape and avoid our problems, the more personal and social damage we cause. You'd think we'd be ready to come to terms with our sick society and face our problems, but nothing could be further from the truth. Rather than getting more honest about our problems with food, drugs, sex, alcohol, gambling, the Internet, and myriad other substances and activities, we've stuck our heads even deeper in the sand.

"What problems?" many ask, oblivious to the current implosion of our society. "What obesity? What gambling addiction? What obsession with sex and pornography?

We won't stand up and own our vulnerable condition. We won't look one another squarely in the face and come clean about our condition. We're just too ashamed, and so we hide.

I recently had lunch with a good friend who hosts a successful television program. He told me that he is discovering that more and more of his faults are open to him and to others. This caught my attention.

"All the things we hide when we're younger come out on the table when we're older," my friend said matter-of-factly.

"Why is that?" I asked.

"I'm not sure, but I know it's true. My theory is that as we get older, we become less inhibited and more likely to act out. If we've struggled with sexual temptation, we may become less inhibited about those temptations. If we've struggled with anger, we may become more crotchety and irritable when older.

"Interesting," I mused. I immediately began to worry about issues I might still be hiding from others and how they could be exposed.

"When we're younger, we tend to think no one will ever discover our secret sins," he continued. "We often think we're invincible. We believe our faults won't catch anyone's attention, but that's not true. The truth has a way of escaping to the surface, sometimes sooner rather than later."

"We feel so much shame," I agreed, "and expend so much energy trying to hide our faults."

"Yes," he concluded, "and when we're older, either we come to terms with those faults and deal with our issues, or other people finally call us on them. I've seen it work both ways."

Humility

Yes, we often build walls around ourselves, keep secrets in and truths out, and live in self-deception. In my professional experience, people wrestle with two extreme viewpoints of themselves: They think they are either worse than they are or better than they are. If we don't let a few trusted people help us understand ourselves, we can become mired in confusion.

The first trap is to think too poorly of yourself. In spite of the recognition you receive and countless positive attributes, your failures loom large in your mind. In fact, all you can see are your failures. When people remind you of your strengths and accomplishments, you find some reason to dismiss them because you feel inferior to others.

Many who struggle with low self-esteem feel particularly crazy. While other people are continuously trying to fill their bucket, the holes in the bottom never allow any of the positive affirmations to build up. Nothing anyone says seems to make a difference to people who have struggled with self-esteem issues their entire life. They perceive themselves as weak, inferior, and prone to failure, and no evidence to the contrary changes their opinion.

The other trap is at the other extreme on the self-esteem scale—that of grandiosity. People who err in this direction are puffed up like the pastor I talked about earlier. They can seemingly do nothing wrong. They are arrogant, prideful, and often condescending. They may seem secure, but they're not. Their bucket has just as many holes in it as the person with obviously low self-esteem. Grandiose people can't be told often enough how wonderful they are. They continually seek compliments and admiration.

If feeling like you are worse than others is not the answer, and feeling better than others offers no more relief, what is the answer? The apostle Paul offers the answer: "Do not think of yourself more highly than you ought, but rather think of yourself with sober judgment, in accordance with the measure of faith God has given you" (Romans 12:3).

Think of yourself with sober judgment—not too high or too low. This is easier said than done, and Paul offers a bit more counsel on the subject. In the next several verses he notes that each of us has been given certain gifts that we are to exercise. In other words, be the person God has called you to be. Follow your gifting. Live according to your unique calling. If you will do this, you will feel God's pleasure and grace.

A primary solution to our problems of feeling shame, hiding, and wondering if we are crazy is to embrace humility. The word *humble* comes from the Latin *humus,* or earth. This doesn't imply being lowly, but being honest and authentic. We are enough just the way we are.

Jesus also gave counsel on this topic. In the Sermon on the Mount, Jesus says, "Blessed are the poor in spirit, for theirs is the kingdom of heaven" (Matthew 5:3). Jesus' teaching suggests we are to be teachable people who are open to new understandings.

Transparency

One of the benefits of counseling is that it offers us a place to be free to be exactly who we are. After all, we surmise, we're paying this person to listen to us regardless of what we talk about.

In a recent counseling session, I met with a young, anxious mother. Karen has been in counseling with me for several months, striving to be a more effective mother. She is a warm, caring woman and has read and practices most of the strategies in Christian parenting books. She describes her two children, aged seven and ten, as being very well-adjusted, but she fears ruining them with one slip of her parenting skills.

Karen came to counseling for help in disciplining her kids. From every description of them, they appear to be bright, well-adjusted, and sociable. They're already learning the Scriptures. You might think Karen would be self-assured. Her parenting skills are fine. But her perfectionism makes her feel anxious nonetheless. Each session has begun much like the previous one.

"Do you think I'm doing OK with my kids?" she'll ask after describing the way she handled a particular situation.

"Yes, Karen," I say. "Your kids sound wonderful. You sound like you're doing a great job."

This is rarely enough reassurance for her. "But you don't know what I did this morning," she says anxiously, preparing to confess an apparently horrible wrongdoing.

"What happened?" I ask.

"Jenny was whining this morning and wouldn't stop. She was dawdling and was going to be late for school. I don't know what came over me, but I started yelling at her. She got even more upset, and I finally grabbed her and told her to get into the car without breakfast. I left her at school on a pretty sour note."

"Yep," I said without much emotion, "sounds like a typical morning for a lot of families."

"I feel like a neglectful parent when I lose my temper with my kids."

"Do you remember Dobson's book on parenting?" I asked.

"Of course. *Parenting Isn't for Cowards.*"

"Do you see the point, Karen? Parenting is not an exact science. It sounds like you actually handled the situation fairly effectively. The yelling wasn't the best, and maybe you could have talked about it on the way to school, but letting Jenny miss breakfast because of her dawdling was an appropriate consequence."

Karen seemed relieved. She is learning that she is a conscientious parent who must loosen her expectations of herself. She strives for perfection, but she must give herself room to be human. She must recognize that she will never be a perfect parent and that all of us parents have failed in some way. She must learn that she is doing enough for her kids, that they will turn out just fine, and that she can relax. Of course, this is often easier said than done.

Karen has joined a support group at her church for parents. She listens to other people who struggle to be effective parents. She is able to be transparent, sharing her triumphs and failures as a parent. It is an important source of comfort for her.

Self-Acceptance

The Bible pictures us as the crowning glory of God's creation, but many of us feel like Karen as our self-esteem teeters on the brink of disaster. In spite of our endless list of accomplishments, we're only one mistake away from feeling like utter and complete failures.

For example, I have a passion for writing, and I've experienced some success. But I still look over my shoulder and wonder if my readers or my publishers will discover that I can't really write and that the success of my books is actually a fluke. I've come to understand that this fragile balance of self-esteem is quite normal. Most people fear being discovered or even accused of being less than they've trumped themselves up to be.

Getting off this teeter-totter feels great. Rather than bouncing from high to low and back to high again, you can jump off this contraption and find a semblance of sanity in something called self-acceptance.

Self-acceptance is that elusive place where we acknowledge that everybody is a bit crazy, but we're not as crazy as we fear. We can smile at our neurotic tendencies and our numerous idiosyncrasies, and still strive to be better. Like the old button said, PBPGINFWMY—Please Be Patient, God Is Not Finished With Me Yet.

Rabbi Irwin Kula tells a delightful story in his book *Yearnings,* illustrating that self-acceptance is one of our most powerful antidotes to feeling crazy. His daughter, Gabriella, was asked on a high school entrance exam, "What makes you unique?" She struggled to answer the question, delaying her answer for days until she had little time left before the assignment was due.

Her parents were mystified. "Gabriella was a developing artist—designing her own line of clothes—and a talented writer. Didn't she see how special she was? Her response blew me away."

The question wasn't so simple to Gabriella. "Yeah, Dad, but lots of people are those things too. And besides, none of it is all of who I am. I'm everything put together, and not even that. There's always new stuff."

After their discussion, Gabriella wrote, "What makes me unique is that I am always Gabriella-ing. No one else in the world does that."[2]

Isn't that the truth? I'm always David-ing, and my wife is forever Christie-ing. No one adjective could possibly capture who I am, who Christie is, or who you are. If I tell you I am a writer who is passionate about helping people and sailing and being with our family and taking long hot tub soaks and reading stories out loud with my wife and sneaking off to discover new cities and bed-and-breakfasts, that would still only be a partial truth. If I added that I can be impulsive and dreamy and energetic and humorous and politically incorrect, that would still be incomplete.

We are made in the image of God, and we have almost limitless possibilities. Just as we can never grasp the infiniteness of God, we can never fully understand or explore the full extent of our possibilities. Our task, however, is to embrace and love all that we discover about ourselves. It includes risking letting others, including God, embrace and love us as well. We drive ourselves crazy when we reject various aspects of ourselves or push ourselves too hard to make sense out of the different aspects of our personality. We will always be becoming, and we can enjoy the ride.

God Only Knows

We may be able to fool some of the people all of the time and all of the people some of the time, but we can't fool all of the people all of the time. And we can't fool God at all, and that's a good thing.

The fact that we can't fool God may cause us to pause and reflect, but can also help us relax. God knows we are in process. He knows we're never as good or as bad as we might think. He knows that we're all trying to be human, that we have emotions and thoughts that seem like a bowl of mixed salad, and that we can make a pretty big mess of things. He loves us nonetheless.

One of the primary goals of this book is to invite you to accept yourself—quirks, idiosyncrasies, and all. This is not an invitation to remain stuck with character traits that need changing but to find that place I like to think of as "being with ourselves." We must companion ourselves on this journey of becoming.

We must remember that none of us have arrived. We are all, like Gabriella, in the process of becoming what we will be, and when we arrive there, we will still continue becoming. Virginia is Virginia-ing, Karen is Karen-ing, and you too are in process. The Scriptures are clear about this process of becoming. Listen to the apostle Paul discuss our spiritual growth process:

> He [gave gifts to men]…to prepare God's people for works of service, so that the body of Christ may be built up until we reach unity in the faith and in knowledge of the Son of God and become mature, attaining to the whole measure of the fullness of Christ. Then we will no longer be infants (Ephesians 4:12-14).

I am so glad God knows my secrets and shortcomings and loves me in spite of them. I am glad He helps me mature. This truth should encourage us to relax and enjoy this process of becoming. We're really not as crazy as we think.

9

But My Family
Is Certifiably Nuts

If you ever start feeling like you have the goofiest, craziest, most dysfunctional family in the world, all you have to do is go to a state fair. Because five minutes at the fair, you'll be going, "You know, we're all right. We are dang near royalty."

JEFF FOXWORTHY

Several months ago, I sat with a teenage girl named Abby and struggled to make sense of her life and her family. Sixteen years old and dressed in jeans and a hooded sweatshirt, Abby slouched in a chair and appeared dazed as she talked about the recent separation of her parents. Staring blankly out the window, she started to cry as she shared her story.

"So what happened?" I asked.

Glancing at me and then back out the window, she began to speak. "My dad's gone. My mom kicked him out. I knew my mom was upset with my dad, but I didn't think this would happen."

"So why did your mom ask your dad to leave?"

Abby took a few moments to answer. "I guess it's my dad's drinking," she said slowly.

"Did you know about your dad's drinking?" I asked.

"No, not really. I knew he went out to the garage every night after dinner, but I never knew why."

"So what led up to your mom asking your dad to leave?" I asked. Abby began to cry harder.

"They had a huge fight the other night. Mom was screaming at Dad, and he was yelling back at her. It scared me. They don't usually fight like that. When I went out to see what was going on, I could tell my dad was drunk. Mom was freaked out."

I waited for Abby to continue.

"I think my mom can't take it anymore. Dad has promised to stop drinking before, but he always starts back up again."

"This has to be very hard for you," I said, sensing Abby's discouragement and sadness.

"I just didn't know," she said, pulling a tissue from the box. "You'd think I would have known my own dad is an alcoholic. But Mom never ever called him an alcoholic until the other night. That's the first time I ever heard her say that."

"Tell me more about what life was like before your mom asked your dad to leave," I said, searching for clues about the dysfunction in their family.

Abby sat quietly, considering the question.

"I'm really confused," she began slowly. "I don't know what to think anymore. If you would have asked me about my family a month ago, I would have said we were normal. But not now."

"What do you mean by that?" I asked.

"Dad was never with us. He was out in the garage drinking. Mom ate, watched television, or played games on the computer. Me and my sisters did our own thing. We never really talked about anything serious. I think we've been avoiding this day for a long time."

"I think so too, Abby. It's very common for families to avoid painful topics. In fact, it's amazing what a family can avoid talking about."

"I hate to admit my dad is an alcoholic," Abby continued slowly. "Some of us are facing things now, but my sister Rachel said she's never coming back home again. I don't think she's interested in talking about this stuff."

"Where is Rachel?"

"She's in college in California. She told me she wanted to get away from our family, but I never really knew what she was talking about until now. I'm starting to figure it out."

The more Abby talked about her family, the more distraught she became. The walls of denial were slowly dissolving. She remembered the earlier separations, when she didn't understand why her dad suddenly left their home. She remembered her parents arguing and her dad angrily peeling out of the driveway as he drove off. She remembered her mom sitting alone in their family room, night after night, depressed. The more she remembered, the sadder she felt.

Abby's father now lives across town in a rented apartment, attending treatment and visiting frequently. Still, her mother is resolved not to take him back until she's convinced of his sobriety. Abby is waiting too, wondering what will become of her family. Her younger sister seems oblivious to the family pain, much as Abby had been oblivious when she was younger. Her older sister remains in California, cynical and resentful, having witnessed even more than Abby. Like her mother, Rachel isn't about to get her hopes up about family reconciliation or her dad's sobriety.

Abby struggles to talk about her pain, unsure of how to explain the confusion, anger, and disillusionment she feels. Abby hasn't learned how to verbalize her feelings about alcohol, abandonment, and neglect. She remains very sad about her parents' separation, her big sister living in California, and her little sister's naïveté about all of it.

Abby is a portrait of her family—fractured, discouraged, and confused. She wonders if she will ever feel normal. She wonders if her family will ever feel normal.

After I talked with Abby, I also talked with her mother and called Rachel. They agreed to a family therapy session. We arranged a time for the entire family to come in and face the critical issues associated with the alcoholism. It was an intervention—a time for the family to start talking about the years of dysfunction.

A quiet sobriety filled the room as Abby and her sisters, mother, and father sat down. Abby's father had prepared an apology, his attempt to begin clearing the air and talking about the problems that had severed his family. He apologized to his daughters and wife and said that leaving the family had been the most painful wake-up call of his life. For the first time in years, the family is truly talking. They are experiencing a hint of normalcy.

It All Starts Here

Abby is a typical adolescent who is searching for answers about her family. Most adolescents struggle to understand why their families act the way they do. They wonder about whom they are becoming and how their family may be shaping that development.

The process of becoming doesn't stop in adolescence. Throughout our lives, we are in process—deciding who we are and who we are becoming. Our journey begins, of course, in our family of origin. That's where we first learn about ourselves, and through the process of genetics and environment, we develop our personality.

Dr. Harriet Lerner, author of *The Dance of Anger*, writes that "family relationships are the most influential in our lives, and the most difficult. It is here that closeness often leads to 'stuckness,' and our efforts to change things only lead to more of the same."[1] Those who are fortunate grow up in families filled with love, stability, strong moral fiber, spiritual values, and a strong dose of healthy genes. Healthy families create security, safety, and a place to experiment with different roles. This is a wonderful environment for a sense of self to emerge. In a safe family, individuals feel a sense of belonging and predictability even if they don't believe in or follow all the family rules. Each member is valued, and the family bestows on each member a sense of worth.

But sometimes the train can slip off the tracks. Good families don't necessarily produce good kids, and some incredible individuals have come from horrific families. Given the variability of these factors, it is easy to lose perspective. If you've attempted to sort out your childhood, you know what I mean. No families are perfect, and a lot of different factors can turn a fairly functional family into a dysfunctional one in a hurry.

Healthy or unhealthy family? Crazy or not crazy? Functional or dysfunctional? Enmeshed, distant, caring, crazymaking? It can be difficult to unravel, and sometimes we feel that our family must take the prize for being the craziest.

If you grew up in a dysfunctional family, chances are you never labeled it that way and never even questioned whether your family was normal or abnormal. Your family is your family. It is everything you know.

At some point you became aware. You reached an age of understanding and began to sit back and reflect on how your family compared to other families. You put things in perspective, much like Abby is doing in her family. You weighed out just how dysfunctional your family was and began making decisions about what to do about it. Stepping back, grabbing a pen and paper, and noting how you were raised and what kind of values you inherited is a valuable experience. You can learn a lot by considering your family of origin and the way it shaped your development.

Dysfunctional and Functional Families

Now of course, the dividing line between crazy and not crazy can be thin and blurred. In fact, as you're beginning to understand, even the word *crazy* has various meanings. But we know what healthy families are like and what unhealthy families are like. We'll consider some of the primary traits that help us distinguish between functional and dysfunctional families. This will help you determine the effect your family of origin has had on you, and it can help you grow beyond any early dysfunction.

1. Does your family talk about problems? Dysfunctional families don't address problems directly or honestly. They avoid issues, just as Abby's family did. A stinky elephant could parade around the home without anyone talking about it. In fact, in severely dysfunctional families, people deny problems exist at all. Denial is a hallmark of unhealthy families. Because of denial, important problems do not get solved.

Functional families talk about problems. They recognize problems, address them, and then work to solve them. They don't keep regurgitating the same issues—they gather, share their perspective on a problem, and then solve it. They create an atmosphere that allows the family to function as a team. Each opinion and perspective is considered vital.

2. Does your family talk about feelings? Dysfunctional families don't talk about feelings. They may have intellectual discussions, but they don't share feelings with one another. They don't know how to identify or label feelings, so they suppress or repress them. But feelings are integral to our identity, so denying our feelings leads to emotional problems.

Functional families talk about feelings. These families recognize not everyone will feel the same way about issues. Family members aren't ridiculed for their feelings or told that their feelings are invalid or unimportant. Everyone's feelings are viewed as sacred.

3. Does your family communicate directly and effectively? Dysfunctional families don't communicate clearly. They don't share their thoughts or feelings, nor do they take responsibility for them. They communicate indirectly through pouting, aggressive outbursts, and passivity. They commit emotional incest by speaking for one another, telling others how they are feeling or what they are thinking.

Functional families practice healthy, direct communication. When family members are upset, they say so. When they experience problems, they talk directly about them. When they are upset at one another, they talk about those concerns. The family members own their own feelings, thoughts, and perspectives, and they are careful to avoid talking for one another.

4. Does your family allow for individuality? Dysfunctional families demand certain behaviors of each other and don't allow for individual preferences. Children are expected to think and act like the parents, and deviations from the family rules incur punishment. Individuality is usually considered selfishness, which is a violation of family rules.

Melody Beattie, in her bestseller *Codependent No More,* reminds us that "the surest way to make ourselves crazy is to get involved in other people's business, and the quickest way to become sane and happy is to tend to our own affairs."[2] Beattie writes about the chaos that ensues when we get overly involved in other people's business, trying to make them see things the way we see them or behave in ways we approve.

Functional families allow for individuality. They recognize that even though the family has clear values, members of the family are individuals. That doesn't give them license to behave any way they want, but they are free to see and feel things in unique ways. Having differences of opinion or personal preferences isn't selfish. It's part of being an individual.

5. Does your family avoid keeping secrets? Dysfunctional families have secrets. They have issues they are ashamed of, and they set up rigid rules and boundaries to keep those secrets safely hidden. Of course, this creates incredible chaos as people worry about keeping these issues secret. And because no one talks about the issues, they don't seek help or experience healing.

In functional families, people share their concerns with each other. They don't have a code of silence. Children are able to talk to their friends, their family, and perhaps even a counselor about what is happening within the family. Everybody is free to reach out to others for support.

6. Can you freely challenge your family's rules? Some dysfunctional families have rigid family rules. There is only one way to do things— the way the family does them. Family members who fail to adhere to these family rules will suffer consequences. People who challenge the beliefs or behavior of the family are criticized and even rejected.

Functional families, in contrast, have flexible rules and allow for the open exchange of ideas. People are allowed to question how things are done and to share their unique point of view. When children ask questions about the family rules, parents listen with an open mind and understand that everyone has his or her own way of viewing things. Everybody's self-esteem grows.

7. Does your family have fun? Dysfunctional families have forgotten how to have fun. Daily life is a serious enterprise and leaves no room for recreation and spontaneous or frivolous activities. Kids in

these families learn not to be too playful or silly. They don't learn how to express humor.

Functional families understand the value of humor and play. They don't take life too seriously. They are able to tease in lighthearted and appropriate ways. They notice the humorous side of life. They understand that laughter is good medicine.

8. Are you safe? Dysfunctional families live with chaos. They have to deal with threats from a tyrannical parent, an alcoholic, a detached parent, or a chaotic "crazymaker." Family members don't enjoy the security of a warm, safe environment, especially when they want to express their feelings, thoughts, or desires. They live in fear, so their self-esteem withers.

In contrast, functional families are safe havens. People are free to express their feelings and thoughts with the confidence that they won't be ridiculed, and they can experiment with different behaviors within reason. People feel accepted, so their self-esteem flourishes.

9. Does your family have moral or spiritual values? Dysfunctional families don't have a moral compass. Without the underpinnings of a moral code, a sense of right and wrong, they are reactionary. They have no road map to guide them in a healthy and functional direction. Consequently, they flounder.

Functional families have a moral compass that guides their behavior and direction. They know right from wrong and are able to instruct, encourage, and confront one another accordingly. Their strong sense of faith helps them stay grounded and clear about how they treat each other and relate to people outside their family.

These are a few of the ways we can determine how functional our families are. Understanding the importance of these traits can lead you into greater freedom and strength.

Family Roles That Bind

Healthy families provide stability and safety for their members. Family members have a sense of belonging, so they can venture out into the world with all its opportunities and dangers and then return home to a place of protection. Nothing feels better than coming home at the end of a rough day to a place where we are safe and loved.

When you think about your family, you probably picture yourself acting in a predictable way. You likely developed a role you performed over and over again. Were you the clown who always made people laugh? Maybe you were the perfect child or caretaker, always frightened of stepping out of line. Maybe you were the rebel or black sheep and tended to choose individuality over conformity. Whatever your role, acting rigidly in a prescribed way is a quick way to feel crazy because after a while, we quit *choosing* to act a certain way and simply play our role because we are *expected* to.

So a family can actually set its members up to feel crazy by expecting them to play certain roles. What is so terrible about family roles? Steven Farmer, author of *Adult Children of Abusive Parents,* explains:

> Whatever role you adopted, it covered up your true self, your Natural Child, behind a false identity. This role has now become a trap that keeps your naturalness and spontaneity buried under an intricate, rigid system of family rules and regulations.[3]

Famed family therapist Virginia Satir, author of *Conjoint Family Therapy,* researched healthy and unhealthy families. She observed five different roles played by family members:

Placaters. Sometimes called caretakers, these people want peace at any price. They dislike anger and will do anything to get rid of it, including pleasing others, apologizing to them, or doing practically anything else to avoid family tension. Sadly, sacrificing themselves in this manner leads to low self-esteem, buried resentment, and loss of individuality.

Blamers. These people are often perfectionists and find fault with others. They accuse other people, attack them, and hide behind their aggressive attitude. They too are trying to compensate for their low self-esteem. They throw guilt onto people who don't live up to their expectations.

Computers. These people are calm and show few feelings. They've learned that they won't be heard or validated, so they suppress uncomfortable emotions. They pretend conflict doesn't exist when it really does, and they hide behind their super-rationality. They too tend to want others to see things their way.

Distracters. Also known as clowns, distracters change the subject to dismiss tension. They may use irrational statements to avoid conflict.

Levelers. Finally, levelers communicate truth through honest feelings, thoughts, and perceptions. They speak their truth without coercing others into thinking the same way they do. They focus on solving problems and promoting cooperation rather than coercion. Our society doesn't encourage leveling because levelers feel vulnerable and transparent.[4]

Roles help us to understand our place in a family, so they help us feel safe and make us feel crazy at the same time. Someplace deep inside we know we're playing a role. We have a sense that we're not being genuine, and keeping up the role requires more and more energy.

Growing up in the Hawkins family was an interesting experience. As the middle of five children, I played the youngest child for several years and then later on played the older brother. I've had ample time to consider the extent to which my family was functional or dysfunctional, crazy or not crazy.

My mother worked as a schoolteacher and my father as a businessman. My father was the son of an alcoholic who died an early death from liver disease. My father learned to cope with life by being a workaholic. Of course, many men who came through the Great Depression and World War II were hard workers. My parents were also fiercely loyal to their church, partly because of their deeply held Christian faith and partly because of the "family" they developed there.

If anything was dysfunctional about our family, it was my parents' intolerance for conflict. Our unspoken motto was "Get along at any cost." This was a close second: "The family must always come first." I learned to hide my anger and unhappiness. My brother had become the placater, and my older sister was the rebel, so I became the distracter or clown. I was always able to find humor in a situation, and I could ease family tension by doing something silly or simply by being loud and obnoxious.

I carried the role well into college before realizing it no longer fit me. I had become such a distracter that I never questioned being anything else. Since then, I have learned about the power of families to reinforce roles, and I can see that I didn't choose this role as much as my family chose it for me. We needed a distracter to ease family tension and restore the equilibrium that was so important to my parents.

What role did you play while growing up? Did you choose it, or did your family choose it for you? Do you still play the role, or have you found a more authentic way to live? Growing out of family roles is challenging work and can sometimes seem impossible. Families press their members into playing roles, and they don't let people out of those roles easily.

Finding your authenticity is important. Identifying the role you play, understanding its value to the family, and then finding your authentic voice are all critical to authentic living. Don't be surprised if you have trouble finding your voice because you've spent years being the child your family needed you to be. Now it's time to decide who you want to be and how to express your newly discovered authenticity.

Our Families' Legacies

Playing roles and living by codes of conduct, even when they aren't completely healthy, are ingredients of the glue that keeps families together. These varied roles also help shape your family's unique identity.

For good and for bad, we each have a family legacy, and our job is to make sense of it. Our family is our most influential context, the main place where we learn about who we are and about the world. Families don't set out to make us feel crazy. They all have underlying tensions, as Harriet Lerner describes in her book *The Dance of Deception*:

> The level of underground anxiety or emotional intensity [in the family] is a function of multiple factors. It reflects the real

stresses that impinge on the family as it moves through the life cycle, and the parents' economic and social resources to deal with these stresses. It also reflects societal stresses and social inequities that affect the family. It reflects the parents' level of maturity and emotional functioning, which includes their connections to their own families of origin and the unresolved emotional issues they bring from this source.[5]

Lerner is saying we will never fully understand some of the emotional issues that impact our families. These include financial and cultural pressures, religious influences, and personality factors. It's a wonder anyone can come out feeling any semblance of normalcy. With this backdrop of tension and anxiety, family members face a huge challenge as they create their own individuality.

Family tension can lead to polarities within families, legalism, and a denial of individual differences. It often pushes parents to extremes of rigid rules and boundaries or no rules and boundaries at all. It leads to addictions, abuse, and a denial of the truth. Most of us spend a good part of our adult lives making sense out of our childhoods, and for good reason.

I am exceedingly grateful for my family. Our rules were overly harsh and rigid, and my parents were too busy too much of the time, but I appreciate my family's cohesiveness. My parents provided a soothing, listening ear more times than I can count as I've navigated the rough waters of adolescence and adulthood. They have offered me spiritual and moral guidance that has been solid ground upon which I could build a life.

Bad Childhood, Good Life

Fortunately, even a bad childhood that includes prescribed roles and dysfunctional patterns of family functioning can be unlearned. It's never too late to have a happy childhood if you're willing to explore how your family has driven you a bit nuts.

Abby and her family are well on their way to healthier ways of relating. They've named the elephant in the house—alcoholism—and are set on a course to heal from it. They are talking. They are truly listening to one another and embracing each other's unique feelings, thoughts, and behaviors.

Abby is beginning to embrace and accept her pent-up feelings and ideas. She is coming alive for the first time in years as she recognizes her abandonment, confusion, and discouragement. She is beginning to understand the ways that being the child of an alcoholic has shaped her identity.

I remember distinctly when I decided to grow up and confront my father. He had been a rigid and harsh disciplinarian, and he continued directing my life well into adulthood. He told me where and how I should work as well as what kinds of cars I should buy, and this led to many explosive interactions. I pulled away, avoiding his controlling nature but also losing the nurturing aspects of his fathering. I wanted to discover a new way of healthy interacting.

Prior to my predetermined date to have our father-son chat, I studied some of Virginia Satir's books, where she outlines the characteristics of healthy family functioning. According to Satir, "five freedoms" comprise healthy family relationships:

1. the freedom to see and hear what is instead of what should be, was, or will be

2. the freedom to say what you feel and think instead of what you should say

3. the freedom to feel what you feel instead of what you ought to feel

4. the freedom to ask for what you want instead of always asking for permission

5. the freedom to take risks on your own behalf instead of always choosing to be secure and never rocking the boat.

I was moved when I first read these freedoms. I had read Virginia Satir's books when I was in graduate school, but now her words struck a personal chord. Could I actually embrace these freedoms? Should I? After significant pondering, I decided the answer to both questions was yes. I prepared to talk with my father about changing the way we interacted, and specifically, how he interacted with me. I would use Satir's words as a basis for our new relationship.

My father is a loving and generous man, but he was also controlling. He had an agenda for how he wanted things to be. He had a way he wanted me to interact with my sisters, and when I became an adult, that violated my boundaries. He wanted me to continue the role of his obedient son, giving little recognition to my new freedom as an adult. He didn't know it, but we were going to change the way we related to one another. He could want anything, but he would no longer dictate the way I behaved. He could hope I would have certain feelings about our family, but he could no longer prescribe them.

I resented my father for years. I developed the habit of barking back at him when I felt controlled. I would react passive-aggressively, avoiding family gatherings or speaking sarcastically to him. I felt guilty for how I treated him, but I also felt resentful for the way he treated me.

The day came for me to talk to my father. I prayed ahead of time, prepared the words I wanted to say, and then shared my heart with him.

"Dad," I began, "I know you love me. I've never doubted that. I know your heart, and it is always for good. But I am no longer a little boy. I have my own thoughts, my own feelings, and my own way of behaving, which doesn't always match your way of doing things. I'm asking you to allow me the freedom to be my own person. I don't want you to tell me how to interact with my sisters. I don't want you to tell me that my feelings are right or wrong. In fact, unless it directly impacts you, I don't want you telling me how to manage my life."

My dad sat and listened. He wanted to jump in several times, but he restrained himself. By this time, I was 30 years old and he was 60, and he recognized the truth of what I was saying. He knew that he had been overbearing and that the time had come for him to quit trying to direct my life.

My dad sat quietly after I finished asking for what I wanted. Then he looked intently at me and responded.

"David, I know you can manage your life. Of all my kids, I have every confidence in your ability to make something of yourself. What you're asking for is reasonable, and I'll try to give it. All I ask is that when I make a mistake, which I'm bound to do, you'll gently remind me. It's not easy learning new tricks when you're an old dog like me."

We smiled, embraced, and moved into a new and exciting phase of what has proven to be a wonderful adult relationship. My dad catches himself when he's tempted to lecture me. I gently caution him when he begins telling me what to do. I practice the five freedoms vigorously, and they are an encouragement to me.

Dr. Laura Schlessinger, in her book *Bad Childhood, Good Life*, encourages the work that I did with my father and that you can do with your parents. She strongly indicates that we don't have to keep interacting with ourselves or our parents the way we did when we were children.

> Many folks just stay stuck in their childhood ugliness for decades, sometimes forever, angry, bitter, self-destructive, depressed, anxious, or generally out of control and way off any positive track. In a way, these folks become career victims, always unhappy, unbelievably demanding of others, a big chip on the shoulder, an even bigger attitude of entitlement, and generally a propensity for spreading ill cheer... While I suppose it is possible to sometimes make the case that a person was so traumatized and at such a vulnerable time in their lives that it became impossible for them ever to be happy or functional, I don't buy it.[6]

If you've been raised in a family that is certifiably nuts, or perhaps a family like mine—happy and healthy, but with a few characteristics that can throw you off course—take heart. As I said earlier, it's never too late to have a happy childhood. You can decide how you want to conduct your life. You can decide to embrace the five freedoms. You can decide who you want to be around and who you want in your own carefully chosen adult "family." It may include your family of origin, and it may not.

As Virginia Satir suggests, you can create an environment of friends and family that appreciates differences, tolerates mistakes, maintains open communication, and keeps its rules flexible. In this atmosphere, love can flourish, and you can be healthy and happy. Lots of people, perhaps including your family, are ready to embrace healthy freedoms.

Overwhelmed, Under Slept, and a Little Bit Tense

Stress is your body's way of saying you haven't worked enough unpaid overtime.

SCOTT ADAMS

I felt as if I was losing my mind. Truly. On a cool March evening, I was working on my doctoral dissertation—for the fortieth time.

I was sick to death of doctoral anything—writing, rewriting, discussing, reviewing, and preparing to defend my dissertation. I was seeing numbers in my fitful sleep, anticipating criticisms in my dreams, and longing for a return to normalcy.

I was working with a doctoral committee of three professors who were overseeing my work. Each had his own idea of the direction I should take in my dissertation. The only reason I was still enthusiastic about the project was that it led to my doctoral degree.

Late that night, long after my family had gone to bed, I was reading the latest critique of my dissertation. The paper was splashed with red ink from one of my professors. The other two committee members thought the writing and research were fine, but this professor wanted it rewritten. You don't argue with your committee members, even if they don't agree with one another.

I had until mid May to complete the dissertation if I wanted to walk for graduation in June. With time speeding up and adrenaline pulsing through my body at increasing speed, I couldn't sleep, I was losing weight, and I feared I would fly apart.

As I sat on our deck and stared into the forest that bordered our property, I began to weep. I had rewritten this dissertation dozens of times. I had listened intently to my professors' concerns and corrected them, only to have new concerns arise. I shared my frustrations with fellow doctoral candidates, and we became convinced of a conspiracy. It went like this:

The professors wanted us to work our brains to death right up to May 15, when they would magically sign off on our dissertations. No amount of correcting, editing, researching, or defending our work would gain approval before May 15. Like rats in a maze, we were to run and run and run, searching for a nonexistent way out. Our only hope was that the rumor was true—everyone was granted the sought-after three signatures just before the deadline.

This real or imagined diabolical plot fueled our antagonism and fear, but it also offered hope. If all hard-working students really were given the three signatures on the eve of May 15, I would be fine. If, however, this perverse scheme was merely the product of our overworked and stressed-out imaginations, I would slave away another five weeks, losing more and more sleep, with no hope of graduating. My life hung in the balance at the mercy of three professors, and they offered no clues of their ultimate decision.

I spent the next five weeks revising revisions and editing edited versions of my dissertation until I was absolutely convinced my work was essentially the same as the first day I turned it in. Gaunt, restless, discouraged, and fearing the loss of both my mind and my degree, I limped across the finish line to May 15, at which point my professors applauded my work and signed off on the last obstacle between me and my doctorate.

I felt overwhelmed by a strange combination of emotions—anger, humiliation, distress, excitement, and relief. Like a bleeding war veteran who hears the battle is over, all I could do was smile and cry and sleep.

My battle was not unique. Every day mothers rise at the crack of dawn and make breakfast for their children while they frantically prepare for another day at the office. Men scramble to accept overtime shifts at work so they can pay the family bills. Exhausted and discouraged, men and women feel overwhelmed, under slept and more than a little tense. All of this makes us feel a little bit crazy.

Stress

My wife, Christie, gets hives and feels as if she's going to itch herself to death. My friend Tom becomes irritable. I lay awake, fretting and fussing about details I can't control.

The culprit is stress.

Years ago we didn't have a name for it, but now we know it's literally killing us. It is one of the primary reasons we feel crazy, and managing it is a primary way for us to regain control of our lives.

Stress is the psychological and physiological response to events that upset our personal balance in some way. We cannot avoid it. But when we are stressed, we cannot carry on with business as usual because our mental, emotional, and physical balance has been upset. When we face a physical or emotional threat, our body's defenses kick into high gear in a rapid and automatic fight-or-flight response.

We have our own ways to respond to threats, but we usually feel uncomfortable and can wonder if we're going crazy. Often we can't think straight, our hearts pound, our muscles tense, and our bodies go on red alert.

Different things cause stress for different people. For example, a high-powered executive may get stressed by having to spend the day walking on the beach. The retired "beach bum" may get stressed after being cooped up in a cabin all day. Our responses to stress are somewhat unique as well. Just as my wife responds to stress by developing hives and I react to stress by feeling anxious, other people have their own assortment of physical maladies.

Cognitive Symptoms	Emotional Symptoms
memory problems	moodiness
indecisiveness	agitation
inability to concentrate	restlessness
trouble thinking clearly	short temper
poor judgment	irritability and impatience
negativity	inability to relax
anxious or racing thoughts	emotional tension
constant worrying	feeling overwhelmed
loss of objectivity	sense of loneliness

Physical Symptoms	Behavioral Symptoms
headaches	eating more or less
muscle tension	sleeping too much or too little
diarrhea or constipation	being isolated
nausea or dizziness	procrastination
insomnia	alcohol or drug abuse
chest pain	nervous habits
weight gain or loss	teeth grinding
skin breakouts	excessive activity
loss of sex drive	overreacting
frequent colds	picking fights[1]

Headaches, rapid heart rate, thoughts swirling in our brains at warp speed—it's all enough to make you feel crazy. Even just a few of the above symptoms is enough to make us feel as if we're losing control of our lives—and in a sense, we are.

The Stress Response

What God intended for good—our flight-or-fight stress response—has become our undoing. It helped us to survive around saber-toothed tigers, but now it kicks into gear when someone cuts us off on the freeway. Anytime our brains sense an approaching threat, our bodies get ready for action. Our hypothalamus and pituitary glands communicate, and our adrenal glands release the true stress hormones—dopamine, epinephrine (also known as adrenaline), norepinephrine (noradrenaline), and especially cortisol.

Cortisol is incredibly helpful when facing imminent danger. Unfortunately, in today's fast-paced world, we've become sensitized to stress, and our bodies pump out far more cortisol than is good for us. Overproduction of adrenaline and cortisol results in obesity, heart disease, osteoporosis, and numerous other physical and emotional problems. High levels of cortisol have even been shown to kill off brain cells that are crucial for memory.

Our bodies are confused. The reaction originally reserved for dangerous situations is now activated in the most mundane circumstances. We're ready for war if we're turned down for a promotion. We're aggravated if our cell phones don't work properly. We're stressed out if we have to wait more than three minutes for a hamburger, and heaven help us if we miss a flight or our cars won't start.

Tragically, we spend far too much time in fight-or-flight mode. Our bodies are screaming for help—we aren't facing life-or-death situations and certainly don't have any saber-toothed tigers to deal with. However, as we become sensitized to the stress response and our bodies release biochemicals, they are slowly killing themselves. The onslaught of biochemicals assaults our immune system, opening the way to cancer, infection, and disease.

The World Is a Stressful Place

I've become a gadget junky. I like my cell phone—actually, a personal digital assistant—laptop computer, and GPS for my car. Unfortunately, I'm no engineer, so every time any one of these instruments goes on the fritz, I'm upset. I get downright irritated.

I want my laptop to work perfectly every time I turn it on. I want my GPS to understand where I want to go and how to get me there.

I want my cell phone to remember everything I put into it, never drop a call, and keep me entertained. I'm not always pleased with the results.

Christie and I absolutely dread going into the local cell phone store to get our phones maintained, repaired, or replaced. We try to pawn the job off onto each other, but we're both too savvy for that, insisting we join forces rather than go in alone. We'd rather walk across hot coals than spend a perfectly good Saturday afternoon dealing with our phones.

Obviously, our attitude could use a little work. We're the ones who've become cell-phone dependent. We're the ones who drop our phones in the toilet or overboard on our sailboat. We're the ones who had to have the phone with the most functions, instead of sticking with the simpler tried-and-true model.

Before even getting to the store, I've practically had an anxiety attack, and Christie has broken out in hives. I imagine the worst-case scenario and discuss it with Christie before even starting our car to drive 50 miles to the nearest dealer.

"We're going to get there at the absolute worst time," I lament. "A hundred customers will be crammed into the tiny store, and three of the four clerks are going to be out sick. Soon as we take a number, we'll get that 'We've got you now, sucker,' feeling, and we won't turn around because we drove fifty miles to get here. All we can do is look at the three hundred different phones and pretend we have a clue about what they do and how they do it."

Christie has only a slightly better attitude when it comes to cell phone purgatory.

"I hate this," she'll mutter. "Why do we do this to ourselves? I knew I should have stuck with my old cell phone. It never caused me any problems."

By this time, her hives are worse, and my breathing has become shallow and forced. I'm focused on negative recurring thoughts about this waste of time and how frustrated I'll probably feel when the deal is done. I'm ready to meet a saber-toothed tiger or fight off invaders to our national security. Of course, we don't meet any tigers—only a thin man with a pocket protector who is talking to customers one at a time and who doesn't deserve my disdainful thoughts.

Christie and I are not alone. Too many of us have created a world that's too stressful. We've become too busy, too intense, and too pressured with too many things on our minds. It's all too much, and it makes us feel crazy.

Edward Hallowell, author of the popular book *CrazyBusy*, believes much of our stress comes from our increasingly busy lives in our increasingly busy world.

> Without intending for it to happen or knowing how it got started, many people now find that they live in a rush they don't want and didn't create, or at least didn't intend to create. If you feel busier now than you've ever been before, and if you wonder if you can keep up this pace much longer, don't feel alone. Most of us feel slightly bewildered, realizing we have more to do than ever—with less time to do it.[2]

Christie brings a bit of balance to our cell phone experience. She slows us down better than I do. In fact, even though she hates the cell phone store as much as I do, she can shift gears and make it a tolerable experience. She reminds me that a Starbucks store is just a few doors down, and we can keep our number at the cell phone store while we grab a latte. Good decision.

Sources of Stress

The cell phone store is not fun for me, but the problem really isn't the store, and I know it. The problem is inside me. For some people, cell phone shopping is an exhilarating experience. One person's stressor is another's joy. This seems inherently odd to me, but it's true. My stressors are unique to my personality.

However, some common attitudes create stress for nearly everyone. These attitudes make everyday stressors, like traffic, busyness, and broken dishwashers, even more stressful. They also make larger stressors, like illness, job loss, and divorce, more stressful as well. When we learn to manage these attitudes and stop allowing them to manage us, we will live less stressful lives.

Uncertainty. Most of us like the familiar. We want our lives to be predictable. We want to know how much money we'll make on our next paycheck. We want to know we can pay our bills, come home at the end of a workday to an orderly house, and enjoy long-lasting health and well-being. In short, we don't like uncertainty and will often create more stress for ourselves by trying to avoid it. The challenge is to embrace uncertainty, recognizing it is an inevitable aspect of life.

Perfectionism. We could avoid many of life's stresses by not trying to micromanage things. We want things to proceed just the way we picture them, and we become stressed out when life throws us a curve ball—which it does with regularity. We must keep a loose rein on our lives so we can adjust to unexpected circumstances. We must not expect too much out of ourselves or others, or the normal disappointments of everyday life will make us inordinately unhappy.

Unrealistic expectations. Like perfectionism, unrealistic expectations set us up to strive too hard, feel too much pressure, and be disappointed. We all want to reach for the stars, but we must keep our sights set on reasonable targets. If we constantly push ourselves to perform, we aren't left with much room for relaxation and rest.

Low self-esteem. When we continually come up short, we feel bad about ourselves, and that feeling is a primary source of stress. If we are always answering to the inner critic, we will feel as if we can't possibly measure up regardless of how much we accomplish. We can counteract this tendency by finding ways to pat ourselves on the back. We must recognize our strengths, acknowledge our gifts, and celebrate small victories. This brings us joy and a sense of satisfaction.

Lack of assertiveness. Poor boundaries are big-time stressors. When we allow others to dictate how we feel or what we do, or when we let others manipulate us, we are much more likely to feel stressed. Fuzzy boundaries keep us in a constant state of chaos, so our stress response remains activated. Mastering the art of assertiveness gives us the confidence we need to be in control of our lives. The fine art of setting and maintaining boundaries regulates our lives and lowers stress.

Lack of emotional balance. Those who would manage their stress must know how to manage their emotions. They understand their emotional makeup and know how to soothe themselves when they're upset. They know how to manage their anger and don't let resentment build up. They know how to name and embrace their emotions, and they can use their emotions for creative change.

Living with a victim mentality. If we feel we're getting a raw deal in life, and if we believe that everyone is to blame except ourselves, we're going to feel stressed out. If other people are to blame for our unhappiness, then our lives are under their control, not ours. If we don't take responsibility for our unhappiness, nothing changes. We're stuck and will continue to live as victims.

Ingratitude. Some researchers say we're not happy because we're not practicing being happy. That thought may make you to shake your head, but I meant exactly what I said. Some of the latest research on lowering stress indicates that we must practice being happy and appreciating all the blessings we have in our lives. Those who are grateful for the gifts in their lives tend to experience less stress than those who take their blessing for granted.

Lack of spiritual grounding. Study after study shows that a clear spiritual faith mediates against anxiety, depression, and stress. Those who believe in God and see Him as the source of their very being fare better in life. Those who accept their limitations and believe that God is limitless are able to put stressors in perspective. Those who feel connected to God feel somewhat confident that the inevitable storms of life will not overwhelm them.

Can you see how crazy you will feel if one or two of these areas are out of balance in your life? Can you see how vulnerable someone will feel if several of these areas are out of balance?

I recently met with a businessman who felt as if his life was whirling out of control. Tim is a 57-year-old accountant with a health crisis that turned into an emotional crisis as well. He is a large man, at least a hundred pounds overweight. When he came to see me for symptoms of agitation and depression, he initially was gruff.

"I don't know why God singled me out to get diabetes," he said angrily. "Like I need that at this point in my life."

"Do you really believe God singled you out, Tim?" I asked.

"How else can I see it? He certainly could have prevented this, but He didn't. God and I aren't on the best of terms right now."

Tim sat on the edge of his chair, staring at me as if I could give him all the answers he needed.

"Besides," he continued, "it's not like that's my only issue. I'm working harder and enjoying it less. My wife says I'm a bear to live with, and I've got to admit she's probably right. I'm just so furious about this diabetes. I hate it."

"What have the doctors told you?"

"They told me what I thought they'd tell me. They lectured me about my weight. I told them it's not easy being overweight and that I didn't want any lectures about it."

"Tim," I said slowly, "I don't know you, but are you always this angry?"

"Sometimes angrier," he said bluntly.

"Well, I can't help but wonder how that impacts your life. And hearing doctors talk about your weight can't be fun, but maybe that has more to do with your diabetes than God does."

Tim shrugged. He spent the rest of our session as well as the next talking about his life and how he felt victimized. Clearly, however, Tim was no victim. If anything, he victimized others. Our list above shows that Tim was at an extreme risk for being stressed out.

> He can't live with uncertainty,
>
> he is perfectionistic about himself and others,
>
> he has unrealistic expectations of others,
>
> he blames others for his problems,

he lacks healthy assertiveness,

he doesn't trust in God,

he lacks emotional balance, and

he lacks gratitude.

I have my work cut out for me, as does Tim. He is a very unhappy man, and the way he deals with stress only makes him unhappier. If he is to manage his depression, he will have to look carefully at the way he deals with his emotions and his attitude. He must stop blaming God for his misfortune and examine his role in it. Specifically, he will have to manage his weight, accept and manage his diabetes, and change his emotional outlook. Anger and resentment will only exacerbate his problems. Finally, he must become grateful for his blessings and explore ways to make his life happier.

Your Stress Vulnerability

When cortisol is pumped into your bloodstream at eye-popping speed, you won't feel more in control of your life, unless of course you are facing that saber-toothed tiger—or a burglar entering your home.

Those are not likely scenarios, so if you want to feel less crazy, you *must* determine to manage your stress. You must name it, claim it, and then maim it. It's yours, unique to you, and you are the only one who can do anything about it. Here are a few factors about stress that will be useful to you.

1. What are the stressors in your life? Specifically, which ones do you have some control over, and which ones are out of your control? Stressors that involve some central aspect to your life, such as your marriage, job, or health, are likely to be experienced as the most stressful.

2. Are you facing a crisis? If something truly is a crisis—something that challenges your resources to handle it—this will obviously be more overwhelming to you. But be careful not to label something a crisis unless it indeed is one. If it is, take measures to effectively manage it.

186 Normal People Do the Craziest Things

3. How do you perceive these stressors? Perception is everything. The way you label the stress in your life shapes the way you will react to it. If you tell yourself that the situation is challenging but manageable, you will fare better than if you tell yourself the situation is devastating.

4. How much do you understand the stressor? The more you know about your stressful situation, the better off you'll be. The more prepared you are, the better. For example, if you are facing a job loss, learn all you can about how to find a new job. If you are facing financial pressures, learn everything you can about how to manage your financial resources.

5. How much confidence do you have in your ability to face stressors? The more confidence you have to face challenges, the better off you'll be. The more you're able to roll with the punches, the less crazy you'll feel when meeting a crisis. Remind yourself that you've handled similar crises in the past and can handle this one now.

6. How much support do you have? Studies repeatedly show that friends and family provide an invaluable buffer against the stressors of life. Having a good friend to talk out problems with can literally be a lifesaver.

After you have accurately assessed the stress in your life and your resources to handle it, take advantage of the many additional tools at your disposal for managing life's challenges. Here are a few additional tools to help you regain control of your life and minimize those feelings of craziness caused by stress.

Stress Busters

Thankfully, you can manage your stress. We create most of the pressures in our lives, and we can minimize them. If we're willing to use the tools in our mental health toolbox, we can find creative and individualized ways to regain our emotional composure.

We must always remember that we're the primary creators of our stress. We are often tempted to blame others or even God, but we're the ones who bring the majority of stress upon ourselves. But this should also give us hope because we can marshal our resources and bring the tiger of stress under control. Here are a few ways to do it.

1. Be proactive in managing stress. Don't wait until you're completely stressed-out to pull out your de-stressing toolbox. Know what calms you and be ready to employ those tactics before your stress is out of control. Understand that what works for others may not work for you. Know what calms you and gives you a sense of inner peace.

2. Avoid quick fixes for reducing stress. Notice whether you tend to reach for fatty foods, alcohol, cigarettes, or other substances that do not reduce stress. Those things actually add to it!

3. Practice spiritual disciplines. The psalmist tells us, "His delight is in the law of the LORD, and on his law he meditates day and night" (Psalm 1:2). Scripture reading and meditation, prayer, fasting, service, solitude and silence, and simplicity are only a few of the de-stressing disciplines available to us. Richard Foster's *Celebration of Discipline,* Dallas Willard's *The Spirit of the Disciplines,* and Richard Dahlstrom's *O_2* are excellent reads on this topic.

4. Slow down. Purposefully slow down your pace. Become mindful of your life and the wonder of God's creation. Take time every day to focus on your breathing. Pay attention to how you are feeling, noting what adds stress to your life, and then endeavor to do something about it.

5. Journal. Taking note (literally) of your life is a proven stress reducer. Choose a journal and pen that feel attractive to you and begin a practice of writing daily about your life. You'll begin to notice patterns and issues that will require even more attention. You can also note people, places, and situations for which you are grateful. Journaling can be a form of contemplation and even prayer.

6. Exercise. This is the great elixir of life because it allows us to drain off excess tension. Exercise is good for you in many ways, including increasing attention, improving mood, and reducing anxiety and stress. If you haven't established a regular pattern of exercise, do it now!

7. Set boundaries. So much of our stress comes from not setting healthy boundaries. We allow others to talk us into situations we'd

rather not be in. We let them manipulate us or aggravate us. Setting healthy boundaries is like maintaining a fence around our minds, protecting our minds from unwanted intruders. We have mental gates that we open to those we trust and close against those who are not safe to us.

8. Relax. You can train your body to relax. This cannot be done in one or two easy steps, but you can learn how to do it. Many people begin with a routine like this: Sit comfortably with your eyes closed, tensing and then relaxing your muscles. Begin with the tips of your toes and move up until you reach the muscles in your face and neck. As you do this, breathe deeply. Place one hand on your abdomen and the other on your chest, breathing in slowly through your nose. Feel your abdomen rise as you breathe deeply. Feel yourself begin to calm.

9. Find time. Many of us are irritated about our busy schedules and are searching for ways to find more time. We want more time to garden, sail, hike, exercise, or simply meet our friends for lunch. We are eager to find a few solitary moments to write, dream, and consider our lives. As Sarah Susanka, author of *The Not So Big Life* says, "There's an amazing amount of wasted space and time in our lives, which, when cleaned out, reveals a lot more room to work with for remodeling. You can think of the process as the psychological equivalent of spring cleaning."[3] Make a decision to create more time in your life to do the things that add pleasure rather than filling it with things that create stress.

10. Create a sense of community. Isolation increases our stress, but knowing that we belong decreases it. Ray Oldenburg, in his book *The Great Good Place,* talks about the "third place." The first place is home, the second is work, and the third is someplace you go to hang out. The third place has now been recognized as a place like the bar on the television show *Cheers,* where everybody knows your name.

Some people might find this third place at their corner coffeehouse, where people go to just chat with friends. Others find it at church. Still others seem to experience this camaraderie at their gym. Cecile Andrews points out in her book *Slow Is Beautiful* that "community is about caring for people, feeling safe, feeling accepted, feeling like you belong."[4]

Don't Worry, Be Happy

It shouldn't surprise us that Jesus talked about stress and offered a remedy for it. Addressing the issue of worry, one of the greatest sources of stress, He said, "Do not worry about your life, what you will eat or drink; or about your body, what you will wear. Is not life more important than food, and the body more important than clothes?"

Then he offers a powerful image for our consideration. "Look at the birds of the air; they do not sow or reap or store away in barns, and yet your heavenly Father feeds them. Are you not much more valuable than they? Who of you by worrying can add a single hour to his life?"

After discussing our propensity to worry, Jesus offers a solution that at first glance seems too simple. "But seek first the kingdom and His righteousness, and all these things will be given to you as well. Therefore do not worry about tomorrow, for tomorrow will worry about itself. Each day has enough trouble of its own" (Matthew 6:25-34).

Jesus' words remind us that we tend to worry too much about things we have little control over. We get bogged down in the details of life, forgetting the more important matters, such as our faith. We forget that we have a heavenly Father who cares for us more than anything and wants our best. This is a fabulous stress-buster and brings the other issues of life into perspective.

Dance of
the Porcupines

*For one human being to love another, that is the work
for which all other work is but preparation.*

RAINER MARIA RILKE

Perhaps the most common place to feel absolutely crazy is in the middle of a relationship. Nothing is quite like being in close proximity to someone, day in and day out, to occasionally make you feel claustrophobic, paranoid, and possibly even schizophrenic.

Why such a harsh depiction of relationships? If you've ever been married or engaged or have dated someone for longer than two months, you know that relating can be very tricky business. Combine your history, replete with its quirks and idiosyncrasies, with another's history, and you've got an interesting combination at best.

Relating is such a challenging situation, social scientists have written thousands of books on the topic, and still we wrestle with one another. Even with endless instructions on how to get along, we make a mess of things as often as not.

If anyone could dance together nicely, you'd think Christians would have it down to an art. We walk with God and talk with God and are filled with His Spirit, so shouldn't we be able to commune with one another peaceably? Apparently the apostle Paul thought so. He repeatedly confronted divided churches and bickering individuals.

Cindy and Cam

I empathized with the apostle Paul the other day as I sat with a couple who came in feeling crazy and left the same way.

"I can't get him to feel sorry for what he's done to me," Cindy said sharply, pointing a finger at her husband during a Marriage Intensive.

She yanked her glasses off and tossed them onto the coffee table. Dabbing at her eyes, she reached angrily for the box of tissue. Cam looked away, rolling his eyes and shaking his head.

"Why are you looking away? You know what you did."

"You'll never let it go, will you? You preach forgiveness, but you hold on like a bulldog," Cam shouted, turning back to her.

"I've loved you in spite of what you did, so you can't say that," she spat back at him. "You can't expect me to just act all loving when you've broken my heart."

"No matter how often I tell you I'm sorry, I can't say it right or act just the right way to pass your inspection."

Cindy and Cam turned away from each other, looking helplessly at me.

I sat quietly for a moment, reflecting on the hundreds of couples I'd worked with over my career. I felt sad and discouraged, and I already wondered about spending two or three hours with their emotional intensity and crazymaking. Why, I wondered, was it so hard for couples to get along? At a time when Cam and Cindy so needed one another, they faced each other as enemies in battle.

Why are we so much like porcupines trying to make love—very carefully? Why, like porcupines, do we prick each other when we try to get close? We can feel so crazy when trying to relate to one another.

"I presume what I'm seeing is why you're here?" I asked. "Is this what it's like at home?"

"Worse!" Cam stated firmly. "We go round and round until one of us gets furious and walks out of the room."

"Do you agree, Cindy?" I asked.

"Yeah. But I think I've got a right to feel the way I do. What Cam isn't telling you is that he had an affair a year ago, and he's never really apologized or made things right."

"That's her version of the story," Cam said angrily. "What she's not saying is how bad things had been in our marriage. What I did was wrong, no question about it. But I was miserable before, and I'm miserable now."

"So it's my fault?" Cindy shouted. "Is that what you're saying? I can't believe this!"

"You see what I mean," Cam said, running his hands through his hair. "I *never* said it was her fault, and I *have* apologized, but it's never good enough. I really don't know what I have to do to put an end to her tirades. We both have a list of complaints. It's not just me who is the bad guy."

"Yes," Cindy screamed at Cam. "Yes, it *is* you who is the bad guy. Don't you think, Dr. David, that I have a right to feel angry about unfaithfulness in marriage?"

"Yes," I said, leaning toward her. "You have reasons to feel bitter and resentful. But scolding him is not going to get these issues resolved. I can't possibly weigh out who has offended whom the most. That's not what I can do for you."

Now both looked at me, sadness hidden in their eyes. There, deep in the recesses of their eyes, were years of pain, sorrow, and disbelief. They never expected to be in this barren place when they signed up for a lifetime of marriage. They could never have imagined the awful words they'd spew at each other in the days, months, and years ahead. Now, illusions gone, they wondered what the future held for them.

"So are we wasting our time?" Cindy asked quietly.

"No," I replied. "As a matter of fact, things can only get better. You've reached the end of your resources, and you're reaching out for help. Thank God, if this pattern is predictable—and it is—then it's preventable. We've got a lot of work cut out for us, but the only way to go is up."

My upbeat response only slowed their pattern of attack for a few moments. It was a long two hours as Cindy and Cam continued finding fault, criticizing, and taking jabs at one another. By the time they left, I felt a bit crazy, I'm sure they felt a bit crazy, and perhaps you're even feeling a little crazy reading about them.

Relationships in Crisis

Cam and Cindy are in crisis. They, like thousands of other couples, face perhaps the greatest challenge they've ever faced. They feel panicky, powerless, and disillusioned about their marriage. All they can see and feel is discouragement. Day in and day out they face criticism, shame, and anger. Like animals caught in a trap, the more they struggle, the worse it gets. The more they rail against their each other, the more acrimony grows.

As we peer into Cindy and Cam's marriage, listening to their harsh and hurtful debate, perhaps you squirm with discomfort. You've probably been there, and so have I. We've been in their shoes, where criticism outweighed compliments. We've experienced the disillusionment that comes naturally when conflict erodes confidence. Will Cindy find a way to forgive Cam? Can they find their way back to loving intimacy?

We've reached a time in history when marriages are ending at alarming rates. Estimates suggest that approximately 50 percent of marriages end in divorce. Many couples will suffer for years in demoralizing, crazymaking conflicts before dissolving their marriages. You may relate to these descriptions of relationships:

Compliments are rare.

Criticism is common.

Verbal battles abound.

Encouragement is nonexistent.

Sarcasm is frequent.

Outbursts are pervasive.

Kindness is elusive.

Discouragement and sadness are familiar.

If this describes your marriage, you're not as crazy as you think. If you've considered divorce, you're in good company. If you wonder about the sacredness of marriage, join the crowd. Relationships are in a state of crisis.

We shouldn't be surprised by this unfortunate state of affairs. Relationships are difficult. Marriages are often turbulent. Ill-equipped and unprepared, many couples enter marriage ready to climb Mt. Everest in tennis shoes. A good marriage is attainable, but approaching marriage problems without the proper tools makes for a difficult climb indeed.

For now, if you're married or in a committed relationship and the sailing isn't smooth, don't abandon ship. Together you can learn some skills that will make the journey much more enjoyable. Before exploring solutions, however, let's examine what makes relating in marriage so much like porcupines making love.

Critical Mistakes in Marriage

Relationships are difficult and can be primary sources for creating feelings of craziness. Anyone who believes relating is simple just may be crazy. Relationships are hard work, and the sooner you understand that, the better.

Fortunately, most mistakes made in relationships can be avoided or at least managed. Most mistakes don't just happen once, but over and over again. And as I told Cam and Cindy, if they are predictable, they are preventable. Together we can begin to understand the predictable mistakes couples make and set out to manage them.

Mountains out of Molehills

In my book *Nine Critical Mistakes Most Couples Make,* I illustrate many of the mistakes I see repeatedly in my practice. One of the most common mistakes I see is the tendency to make mountains out of molehills. It was painful to watch Cindy and Cam bring up what could have been small issues and let them escalate into huge ones. I watched helplessly as they tore one another apart, all the while each one sanctimoniously claiming to be the innocent party. Feeling safe because they saw themselves as victims, they volleyed hurtful barb after hurtful barb, damaging their fragile alliance.

Tragically, escalated barbs often lead one to finally push the plunger and detonate a disastrous explosion. Someone shouts obscenities, slams the door, and stomps off mad. Hurt feelings and wounded egos are left in the aftermath of such an eruption.

John Bradshaw, author of *Healing the Shame That Binds You,* unveils the motivation behind interactions like this. "Criticism and blame are perhaps the most common ways that shame is interpersonally transferred. If I feel put down and humiliated, I can reduce this feeling by criticizing and blaming someone else."[1] These behaviors, explains Bradshaw, lead to feelings of shame, contempt, and rage. Marriages are not likely to survive in this environment.

Cindy and Cam aren't the only ones feeling crazy while snapping at one another. You know the routine. You're tired, hungry, and irritable from a long day at work. You walk in the door, and your mate says something that annoys you. You might have ignored the comment eight hours ago, but now you light into her, snapping at her like an angry crocodile, saying something hurtful. She's hurt and defensive, so she bites back. The battle has begun, and it's not likely to end until someone stomps out of the room.

After a restless night's sleep, possibly alone, you look back on the incident. It was over such a trivial matter, you wonder why you let her comment get to you. You also wonder why you let your pride stop you from apologizing quickly. Now you've got some repair work to do. Making mountains out of molehills makes us feel crazy, and yet it is one of the most common destructive patterns in marriage.

Molehills out of Mountains

Another common mistake leaving us feeling crazy is making molehills out of mountains.

I've told the story elsewhere of the couple who came to see me because of the husband's rampant gambling addiction. The wife was at her wit's end, so she insisted they seek counseling. Midway through the first session, however, just when I was making the case for an intervention that would alter the path of his addiction, applauding her for courageously facing this huge problem, the wife looked at me like I had three eyes.

"Oh, I'm not sure it's that big of a problem," she said. "Actually, I don't think we need to come back. He's only gambling a few times a week, and he's staying within the limits of what we agreed he could spend."

I couldn't believe my ears. He had drained their bank account, racked up thousands of dollars in debt on numerous credit cards, and lied to her and to me. Still she was frightened of facing the problem head-on. They would need to experience more pain and chaos before either was willing to change.

Speaking Unclearly

Another crazymaking mistake is speaking unclearly to one another. Couples typically fight in ways that lead to more fighting. No one speaks clearly because each seeks ways to one-up the other. We complain, bicker, and pummel each other with sarcasm. We don't build one another up, as the Scriptures implore us to do (Ephesians 4:29), but rather put one another down. We talk in circles, jumping from one topic to another, engaging in "pinball conversations." We don't seek solutions and rarely stumble upon them.

The solution is to speak clearly, stating exactly what you feel, think, and want, always carefully owning your feelings and thoughts and never speaking for your mate. Clarity is the hallmark of healthy communication.

Playing God

Couples also get into real trouble when they make the mistake of playing God. The apostle Paul admonishes us not to think more highly of ourselves than we ought (Romans 12:3). Thinking we know all of our mate's faults, we do incredible damage by telling each other what to feel, think, and do. We arrogantly play God, exaggerating our own importance, putting our mate down, and making him or her feel inadequate.

Criticism

As if putting our mate down isn't enough, many couples make another crazymaking mistake and criticize one another. They battle it out in the trenches rather than cheering for each other in the grandstands. Here's the difference:

- You forget to compliment your mate.
- You disregard what is important to your mate.
- You make sarcastic comments.
- You voice uninvited criticisms freely.
- You live a humdrum existence.

We are all hungry for consideration. We want someone to ask us about our day. We want to look forward to special events. We want to know that someone cares about what is important to us.

Couples who live in the grandstands enjoy weekly dates. They never lose sight of why they married each other, and they share their love freely and frequently. They keep the romantic spark alive.

Violating Boundaries

Many couples make the mistake of violating one another's boundaries, creating real chaos. We allow others to invade us, especially our mate. In fact, we often have little awareness of how others hurt us. We know we're being hurt, and have a sense that something toxic is taking place, but we don't know how it is happening or how to stop it. Sue Patton Thoele suggests this in her book *The Courage to Be Yourself*:

We become vulnerable to invasion through fear: fear of rejection, imperfection, embarrassment, or confrontation. Because we fear other people's reactions, we allow them to violate our limits and boundaries. Fortunately, our physical and emotional responses tell us when someone has trespassed on our private selves, and we can learn to tune into those feelings and use them as valuable clues for maintaining reasonable limits.[2]

Thankfully, it's never too late to begin learning the fine art of setting boundaries, and a marriage is an excellent place to practice these skills. Setting healthy boundaries is a tremendous way to feel less chaos and craziness in our lives.

An Untamed Tongue

Perhaps nothing makes us feel crazier than listening to an untamed tongue. On a recent outing to Safeco Field to watch the Seattle Mariners, Christie and I sat behind a couple who spent more time bickering with one another than watching the game. We tried not to be distracted by their banter, but it was hard not to eavesdrop.

She nitpicked him for not getting some errands done. He railed back at her for being too lazy to do them herself, because she wasn't working that day. She countered defensively that he had agreed to do them.

The couple continued accusing one another, casting blame in large doses until they finally settled into a resentful silence, watching the remainder of the game. We were thankful they had given up the fight, but we couldn't help feeling saddened at how they mistreated one another. Although we both hoped what we saw was an aberration, I suspect they pick at each other like this regularly.

The apostle James laments about the untamed tongue, likening the tongue to a spark that can set a forest ablaze: "The tongue is also a fire, a world of evil among the parts of the body. It corrupts the whole person, sets the whole course of his life on fire, and is itself set on fire by hell" (James 3:6).

We must recognize that harsh words can never be taken back. Hurtful comments cut deep, bruising not only the ego but also the soul of your mate. Take care never to use words that will set your relationship on a downhill slide.

Distance

Possibly the greatest crazymaking mistake we can make is being distant. This final critical mistake has to do with intimacy, or "into me see." Many couples live parallel lives, never quarreling and never talking substantially either. They live in different worlds. She learns to busy herself with the children while he spends his energies building a career, saving a little room for a round of golf on Saturday. Evenings are spent in front of the television, and their marriage begins a slow death.

Countless couples come to me after years of being distant with only a few dying embers remaining in their relationship. Some are fortunate enough to rekindle the flame; others are not. How vibrant is your marriage? How close do you feel to your mate? Is it time to take inventory and resolve to re-create your relationship?

Power Struggles

The apostle James had more to say about relationships, especially why they fail and make us feel crazy. In a most telling portion of Scripture, James asks a piercing question.

> What causes quarrels and fights among you? Don't they come from your desires that battle within you? You want something but don't get it. You kill and covet, but you cannot have what you want. You quarrel and fight (James 4:1-2).

James seems to have been sitting in the corner of my office, watching me interact with my clients. He must have witnessed the endless stream of couples begging for help, only to turn on one another like cannibals.

James talks straight to us. We want what we don't have, so we fight and quarrel, trying to coerce our mate into agreeing with our point of view. We try to bully them into thinking the way we want them to think and feeling the way we want them to feel. Ultimately, we want our mate to do what we want them to do. We don't want our mate to be free-thinking, unique individuals. We want them to be a clone of us.

The irony is that all our maneuvering doesn't change our mate—it actually makes them retreat and resist us. How many people change after being badgered to death? Not many. How many want to cooperate after being browbeaten into submission? Coercion, manipulation, and power plays only breed resentment.

Unsuccessful in our manipulative endeavors, we pout, whine, throw temper tantrums, and sometimes even become violent. We stop at little to get our way. No wonder we feel broken and discouraged in marriage! Can we really blame our mate for wanting to get away from us at times? After all, we're not as easy to get along with as we'd like to imagine.

Rosamund Stone Zander and Benjamin Zander wrote a fabulous book that can help us break out of these win-lose power struggles that are so rampant in relationships. In *The Art of Possibility*, the Zanders describe our two natures and the way they war with one another. The Zanders discuss the *calculating self,* which is designed to look out for number one. We will stop at nothing to get our way, setting up win-lose scenarios. The calculating self sees the world as being small, with not enough to go around. "Get yours before someone else gets it," it says.

There is another way: The *central self* is generative, prolific, compassionate, and creative. It seeks other people's welfare. Living from our central self, we give up taking ourselves so seriously. We're willing to ask for forgiveness, appreciating our mate and their well-being. "When one person peels away layers of opinion, entitlement, pride, and inflated self-description, others instantly feel the connection."[3]

These words may sound familiar. They can be found in a varied form in the Gospels, where Jesus tells us, "If you try to hang on to your life, you will lose it. But if you give up your life for my sake, you will save it. And what do you benefit if you gain the whole world but lose your soul?" (Matthew 16:25-26 NLT).

Those last words are so indicting. What do you gain if your calculating self can manipulate others into submission—a mate who cowers and caters to your every demand? You win her submission but lose your soul and the soul of your marriage. Obviously, this is not the answer. Small, calculating, frightened relationships are not rewarding. Caring for the welfare of your mate brings satisfaction. Being a servant is far more gratifying than demanding slavery.

Appreciating Our Differences

We're all a little bit crazy, and the sooner we realize that and accept it, the better off we'll be. We all have quirks and idiosyncrasies that take some getting used to. Some of us are introverts, and some are extroverts. Some are neatniks, and others are slobs. Some love the outdoors, and others prefer watching Mother Nature from an air-conditioned distance. On our journey of realizing we're not as crazy as we think, one of our tasks is to notice these differences and realize they need not be divisive. When we walk through a zoo or an aquarium, we see different animals. Yes, some are cuter than others, but each has its important place in the ecosystem.

Once we realize that we have differences and accept and appreciate them, we can get on with the task of relating to each other. We can let go of comparisons and divisive notions, such as "You are smarter than me," "I am stronger than you," or "I am sicker than you." When we allow our differences to drop into the background and we bring our commonalities to the foreground, we open the door to intimacy and contact.

Just yesterday I talked on the phone with Daniel, who is experiencing a crisis. Tearfully he told me his pastor had referred him to me in a last-ditch, desperate attempt to save his marriage. "I can't believe it's come to this," he said woefully. "I should have sought help a long time ago. I thought we could fix things ourselves."

"What happened?" I asked.

"My wife felt smothered in our marriage and finally left me. She told me I wasn't giving her room to breathe."

"Did you see this coming?" I asked. "Did your wife let you know there were problems?" I asked.

"Oh yeah," he said sadly, letting out a sigh. "She warned me many times that I was being controlling, but I kept thinking it was her fault. I thought getting help meant I wasn't being strong."

"Everybody needs to reach out for help sometime," I suggested. "Maybe it's not too late. Let's get together and talk about what's happening."

"Great," he said with a faint hope. "I hope we can find a way to turn this around."

Daniel didn't realize that most of us need professional psychological help at some point in our lives. Stress, marriage issues, problems with our children, and any number of other crises can overwhelm us.

I talked for a few more minutes with Daniel. He shared that he couldn't tolerate some of the changes taking place with his wife. With their children grown, he struggled to accept her new desire to go back to work. He felt threatened by her wanting to see her friends. He didn't like her changing attitudes. He acknowledged that he hadn't done well with these changes and that he tended to try to control her, which only pushed her further away.

Navigating differences is one of our most important tasks in marriage and friendship. Differences can deepen our interest and create opportunities, but we tend to be threatened by them and allow them to cause division. Training ourselves to see differences in a new way is challenging. Mastering the art of acceptance and learning to appreciate differences can mean the difference between an exciting relationship and one filled with tension and conflict.

I hadn't yet met Daniel or his wife, but his brief recounting of events suggested what I've seen hundreds of times before: One partner feels smothered and unable to stretch and grow. Expected to remain the same and feeling stifled, she finally rebels and explodes.

Relating is a dance with many subtle moves. In the best marriages, couples learn to anticipate each other's motions. They leave some space between them so each person can change and grow. As the poet Kahlil Gibran said, "Let there be spaces in your togetherness." These spaces afford us the breathing room we need to continue exploring who we really are, a process that lasts for a lifetime.

Daniel may be learning this lesson too late. Feeling stifled and controlled, his wife broke away from his grip. Now he has to learn to let her dance, breathe, and consider whether she will allow him another chance. If she offered him another opportunity, he must be careful to appreciate how she is different from him and how their life together is different than it was before.

Opportunities to Love

The Chinese word for *crisis* combines characters that mean "danger" and "the crucial point." This porcupine dance with our mate can be dangerous because it can lead to conflict and distance. But learning this dance is crucial if we are to avoid feeling crazy.

We often face the risk of pushing too far apart. Each season in a marriage includes critical decisions for us to make. Will we encourage growth in our mate or stifle it? Will we allow our mate the breathing room they need to become who they were meant to become, or will we act critically, soberly, and discouragingly? Will we celebrate our mate and their difference from us?

Michael Gurian tells the story in his book *Love's Journey* about a youthful caterpillar who went around bragging, "When I grow up, I'm going to turn into something else." She bragged to the snail about this, then to the turtle, and then to the polliwog. The polliwog in turn felt sad. "I won't turn into anything," he mourned.

Encountering a fish, he expressed his sadness. "Don't worry," said the fish. "You too will be transformed into something else."

When the caterpillar heard this exciting news about the polliwog, she couldn't imagine the polliwog turning into a butterfly. All the caterpillar knew was that when you turned into something else, it was a butterfly.

The caterpillar and polliwog agreed that the caterpillar would go first in the change process. She set about making a cocoon, spinning till only her head remained unwrapped. "I have to close the lid," she said, "and when I come out, I'll be a butterfly."

Days and weeks went by while the polliwog waited patiently. Suddenly one day, the cocoon stirred. Out came a beautiful butterfly. The polliwog, excited, jumped up and down like a frog. A frog! When had this occurred? He looked himself over. He had become transformed into a frog. "I was so busy watching you," he said, "I didn't notice what was happening to me!"[4]

I've had a similar experience over the past two years. At age 50, Christie decided to finish her bachelor's degree in interior design. A reluctant student, Christie was never convinced this was the right path for her. Yet she persisted, sensing the importance of finishing something she'd started years earlier. She groused about having to take math again after a 20-year hiatus. What possible use could quadratic equations be to her now?

I watched as she put her nose to the grindstone learning computer-aided drawing, often struggling to make the computer perform to her will. I watched her spend late evening after late evening bent over her renderings until she was satisfied.

Awkward and angry, she initially struggled with her classes. On some afternoons and evenings, she wasn't emotionally available to me, and I had to decide whether I would comfort and support her or grouse about feeling rejected. I had to follow the counsel I'd given to hundreds of others—to let there be spaces in our togetherness and to love her into her transformation.

Ever so slowly, her drawings became more sophisticated. Her color boards took on life, her models became possibilities, and her confidence exploded. What was happening here? Christie the student was becoming Christie the interior designer right before my eyes. Last week she graduated with a bachelor's of fine arts—with high honors. And I was proud!

But Christie wasn't the only one transformed. While she was in her cocoon, turning into an interior designer, I had been in my own process of transformation. I had proven something valuable to myself and Christie. I had grown from a self-centered man to someone who could put his immediate needs aside in favor of love. I discovered I could love her, cherish her, and allow her the space she needed to become who she was meant to become.

Scott Peck writes in *The Road Less Traveled* that love means extending yourself for the welfare of another. Extending yourself means just that—pushing yourself beyond your comfort zone in order to meet your mate's needs. Love was never intended to be easy or simple. Transformation is work, and we must provide an environment where our mate can do their work. In return, they will usually do the same for us.

God's Truth About Marriage

Many relationships are in crisis. I won't minimize Cindy and Cam's frustration or the severity of Dan's situation. Yet this is also a time to keep things in perspective. Yes, many marriages are in distress, but many others aren't, and in spite of the challenges, marriage still offers many benefits. It is still a place where we can learn to love.

In *The Case for Marriage: Why Married People are Happier, Healthier, and Better Off Financially,* Linda Waite and Maggie Gallagher offer a counterpoint to all the grousing that takes place about marriage. Instead of rehearsing the old saw that marriage is a stultifying institution, the authors review massive amounts of research to point out the health and financial benefits of marriage.

Marriage, these authors suggest, is good in and of itself. The Bible also offers good reasons for being married, but Waite and Gallagher make a compelling nonreligious case for marriage, noting that married people tend to live longer and have healthier lives. They are generally happier and report greater satisfaction with their sexual lives. They make more money than singles and are happier in their employment. Their children are happier and healthier than their single counterparts.

The authors are quick to point out that simply living together does not offer the most benefits. They note that the legal commitment carries its own benefits as well. The safety and security of commitment to one another brings added benefits.[5]

So even though we're a little bit crazy, we must face the obvious: Marriage was designed by God, and it is good. Now we even have statistical confirmation. God said that it wasn't good for man to be alone, and He instituted marriage. He ordained that we should complement one another, so we should appreciate our differences and not demand similarity. We have an opportunity to provide a safe environment for building cocoons. We can be there when our mate emerges, championing their transformation.

12

Now You See Me,
Now You Don't

*By the time a man is 35 he knows that the images of
the right man, the tough man, the true man, which he
received in high school, do not work in life.*

ROBERT BLY

We are often perplexed by the way our behavior doesn't always match our beliefs. Even the apostle Paul seemed to feel crazy because of this: "I don't really understand myself," he said, seeming to be confused by his behavior. "For I want to do what is right, but I don't do it. Instead, I do what I hate" (Romans 7:15 NLT).

Can you empathize with Paul's confusion and frustration? I certainly can. I often know what I want to do and even intend to do it but don't. At other times, I'm moving full steam ahead on some project, only to find that it's not as rewarding as I had imagined.

Worse yet, sometimes I say things that are hurtful and argumentative, pushing people away, when what I really want is to be close to them. The many different parts of our personalities can create confusion and feelings of craziness. Such was the case with a couple I worked with recently.

"She'll never let you know how depressed and angry she is," Hank said. "You don't have a clue."

I had just completed a weekend Marriage Intensive with Hank and Madeline. Now they were consulting with me by phone, and I thought I knew them fairly well. His words took me by surprise.

Experiencing an empty nest, with their two children now off to college, as well as the normal biological changes that come from midlife, Madeline and Hank suddenly found themselves in a marital crisis. They had flown in from Chicago in a last-ditch effort to save their marriage.

Madeline was a bright, outgoing, and successful Realtor, and Hank was an engineer with a bioengineering firm. She was flamboyant; he was conservative. Both were friendly and worked hard during our counseling, yet the recent months of tension were evident in their subtly biting words to each other.

"What do you mean?" I now asked Hank. "Madeline seemed open and honest to me. You're saying that she fooled me?"

"I don't know about that, Doc," Hank said pointedly. "Let's just say that she's an incredible actress. When we're out with friends, no one knows how angry and depressive she is. She acts sweet and nice to me. But back at home—whew!"

Madeline did seem intense at times during our work together. She was an attractive woman who had a strong and spirited vocabulary. She was critical and logical, demanding that Hank defend his actions.

Hank wasn't nearly as aggressive, tending to be more reserved and thoughtful. He'd often sink into his chair and avoid her questioning. Rolling his eyes in disgust, he shot back short volleys of sarcasm when he disagreed with her. Now, one on one, he was more open.

"I never know who I'm dealing with—the nice Madeline or the one who's going to attack me and find something wrong with everything I do. I'm calling because we've slipped back into all our old ways. I'm having a little trouble thinking straight."

"Tell me what's going on."

"Well, for example, you talked about using the plutonium box. I asked Madeline to leave the issue alone until we could meet with you, but she said, 'Oh, so now we're going to wait until we see Dr. David for anything we talk about? That's handy for you.' Of course, I take the bait and start to defend myself. I tell her we're supposed to call a time-out when things get hot, and she accuses me of never getting around to anything."

"Does Madeline have a point?" I asked.

"I'll admit," Hank said slowly, "I used to be afraid to talk about anything with her. She's brutal, man. She can be nastier than you could ever imagine. But I'm trying to get back to issues. I'm telling you, it's not safe. I'm going to get yelled at and ridiculed, though she'll never admit it. I don't know which Madeline she'll be, and I can't take it."

Hank sounded extremely discouraged. Having dealt with Madeline, I knew she felt equally discouraged, telling me that Hank would rather walk across hot coals than talk about anything emotional. Madeline was caught in a vicious cycle. When Hank retreated, she felt frightened and responded with an attack. But the more she attacked, the more he retreated.

Hank sounded more and more frightened and discouraged as he talked. He shared about his temptation to move out and give up on his marriage. In fact, he'd spent a recent afternoon looking at apartments because he thought they would never be able to resolve their issues.

Many Facets of Personality

Hank implied that Madeline had a split personality. Does she really have these different faces? Is she really two, three, or even four different people? Yes and no.

We all have lots of different facets to our personality. Each of us is capable of doing what Hank accuses Madeline of doing. If we're not careful, we can get confused about which face we're showing to whom. We must be careful that we don't begin to believe we are one part of our personality and not another. This can make everybody feel crazy—us and the people we relate to.

Clearly we act in certain ways with certain people. For example, when I talked with Madeline alone, she was congenial, sad, and discouraged about the way Hank treated her concerns. She felt that Hank talked down to her, dismissing her feelings. She exuded an underlying tone of anger, but she was clear and concise with her concerns. "All I want him to do is listen to me," she had said recently. "I'm not asking him to fix everything. I want him to sit with me, hear me out, and sympathize with my frustrations."

Madeline went on to explain that she felt manipulated by Hank's reserved nature. She complained that he could outwait her, leaving her to stew in her volatile emotions.

Hank, on the other hand, felt manipulated by Madeline's emotionality and insistence that he see things the way she saw them. "If I don't agree with her," Hank blurted, "there's heck to pay. I want the woman I fell in love with, not this bitter woman who comes at me like a snake."

Madeline is a highly successful businesswoman and is able to interact effectively with many different kinds of people. That takes skill and interpersonal effectiveness.

We may feel a bit crazy when our mate acts different ways at different times and with different people, but we must understand that this is normal. In fact it can be a very good thing. Let me use myself as an illustration.

I am normally a cheerful, happy individual. I have a good life with a tremendous wife and wonderful grown children. I live in a beautiful part of the country and enjoy sailing and walking the beach. If you met me, you'd probably like me. However, Christie sees several other sides to me, and these are valid aspects to my personality.

The grump. Christie sees me when I've had a long day at the office and I come dragging into the house out of gas. If she makes any demands on me (which she's allowed to do because of our marriage), I may become grumpy and irritable. I'm capable of grousing about her requests.

The discouraged guy. Even though I'm normally happy, I can get discouraged about some of the typical challenges that come our way. When finances are tight, I've been known to mutter, "As hard as I work and there's no money left over for any fun." Christie has felt unfairly cautious about coming to me with financial concerns because of my discouraged temperament.

The jokester. When I'm in a good mood, which is frequently, I might tease excessively. I can make people laugh, but I've hurt people's feelings by my insensitive teasing. I want others to be sensitive to my feelings, but I'm capable of being insensitive to theirs.

The compulsive worker. A part of my personality becomes obsessed with finishing a task. This is often a helpful trait, but I have been known to lose sight of day-to-day joys, obsessing about the tasks needing to be finished. All work and no play have made David a dull boy more than once or twice.

The selfish guy. I'm often blessed with an abundance of energy and ideas, but I'm prone to forget about other people's needs, like my wife's. I can easily become absorbed in my latest, greatest plans and lose sight of what is important to her.

These are only a few of the different facets to my personality. If you were to call me selfish, that would be true. If you were to call me egotistical, that also would be true. But those are not the entirety of my personality. It would be equally true to call me sensitive, playful, caring, goal-oriented, spiritual, and genuinely nice. I am all of these things—all at once.

I am different around different people. I am most "like myself" when I'm with my wife, who sees all these different aspects to my personality and accepts me. In different situations she is able to see my moods change, my mannerisms change, and even my viewpoints change. I am a complex person; so are you, and so is your mate. You have many facets to your personality, you can act differently in various situations, and you can even lose track at times of what you think and who you really are. Such is the nature of our complex personalities.

So our multifaceted personalities are breeding grounds for feelings of craziness. If we're not careful, we can be overly critical of these different facets. Accepting others and ourselves is very important.

The Shadow

With all of our different facets, we can easily lose track of ourselves. Like the apostle Paul, our actions and feelings can confuse us. One of the explanations for this confusion concerns our "shadow," a concept developed by Swiss psychiatrist Carl Jung.

Jung theorized that the strengths and weaknesses hidden in the recesses of our minds play different roles in the way we act. If we're not conscious of our strengths and our weaknesses, our weaknesses can sneak up on us and cause problems. When I'm not aware of my angry side, for example, I become argumentative without my awareness. If I disown my sadness, I soon feel gloomy and out of sorts.

We are not proud of our weaknesses, so rather than looking at them, we tend to push them out of our consciousness. I don't like to think about my tendencies to joke too much, overwhelm people with my enthusiasm, or pout. I'd much rather think about how adorable I am, my contagious excitement, and my overall good humor and moods. I want to focus on my strengths, and I would rather you see me that way too.

However, the truth is the truth. We all have aspects of our personality that embarrass us. You know the parts of yourself that you would rather ignore or deny. You've got them, and so do I. The problem is that when we deny our shadow traits, they remain outside our awareness and control us.

For example, Madeline is a logical thinker and wants her husband to completely understand her and her problems. She wants every problem solved—now! She has little idea of the overwhelming nature of her emotionality, and she believes Hank's pushing away from her is his problem. She says, "Hank doesn't really care about what's important to me."

This is actually not the case. In my phone consultation with Hank, he reassured me that he is listening to Madeline. He just can't tolerate her lectures. He doesn't want to be reminded of multiple problems at once, and he needs information in small chunks. He is willing to sit with Madeline's concerns, but he needs her to listen to his frustrations too.

Shadow work involves several steps:

1. Realize that you have aspects of your personality that are hidden to you. We all do. Other people can often see things about you that you'd rather not see. You may pretend to be the perfect person, but

others know you're not. You may glory in your strengths while your shadow side is playing havoc in your relationships.

2. Recognize these hidden shadow parts of your personality. We have all been hurt, and we have learned to hide these hurt and ashamed parts of ourselves so we don't get hurt again. These hidden parts are usually filled with anger, sadness, resentment, and sometimes even more pleasant emotions, such as joy.

3. Be aware that these hidden traits can be self-destructive. We've blocked these parts of our personality from our awareness for a reason—they have caused us pain. But denying them and trying to suppress them from our awareness will not help us. These traits will sneak up on us and bite us in the rear. They will continue to play havoc on us.

4. Be willing to honestly observe these traits so they can be healed and transformed. If we are to change and grow, we must bring these troubling traits out of the shadows and into the healing light of God's presence and our awareness. We must courageously invite God to transform us and trust that we can deal with these issues.

5. Believe that your shadow side contains the possibility of transforming weaknesses into strengths. Our greatest strength often becomes our greatest weakness, and our greatest weakness can be our greatest strength. As the Lord said to the apostle Paul, "My grace is all you need. My power works best in weakness" (2 Corinthians 12:9 NLT).

6. Finally, believe that you can heal and transform these traits. With God's help, we can embrace our issues and grow up. We can integrate these fragmented aspects of our personality. We can lovingly accept that we are not perfect and never will be. Additionally, we can discover others are not perfect either, and they never will be.

Robert Bly, in his book *A Little Book on the Human Shadow,* says we are born with "a 360 degree personality," expressing as infants the full breadth of our human nature. Through trauma and development, we learn to censor various disagreeable aspects, only to have them surface in unexpected ways. Many of us are carrying around sacks filled with these disagreeable qualities, thoughts, and impulses. They are detached but not understood and certainly not transformed.

Fortunately, there is gold in the landscape of our shadow side. We can mine our shadow and integrate these various hidden aspects of our personality. This is a sure path to feeling a little less crazy.

Moods

One of the surest signs of our shadow is our moods—stuff that really makes us feel crazy. Not much can make us feel crazier than the moods that sweep over us, often at inopportune times.

We're all familiar with moods. When we say, "I'm in a really good mood," or "I'm in a really bad mood," what do we really mean?

Let's review what we learned about moods in chapter 6 and expand on those thoughts. Usually, a bad mood reveals that we've succumbed to negative thoughts and feelings that make us feel discouraged or perhaps even depressed. We are buried in a mountain of troubling feelings with little hope in sight. Sometimes these temporary moments of insanity last only a few minutes, but for some people they last for hours and even days.

Bad moods can make us feel crazy. Just an hour ago I snapped at Christie for a small problem. I even abruptly walked away from her in anger. I'm not prone to snapping at her or walking away from her, and she would be justified to wonder, *Who is this person who just snapped at me? I don't know him. He looks like David, but he sure doesn't sound like David.*

Sadly, she's seen this snapping person before, so she has a small degree of familiarity with him. I'm sure she would say she doesn't like him, and she certainly doesn't like being snapped at. I don't like him either. Just who is this snapping person?

Now that I've had an hour to think about why I snapped at her and rudely walked away, I've come up with an explanation for what happened. It doesn't justify what I did, but it helps me understand my actions so I can integrate and transform them. In short, I snapped at her because I felt...

angry

misunderstood

discouraged

irritated

unfairly accused

As I grovel, allow me to explain my feelings and what led up to my actions. In my defense, I was experiencing temporary insanity, something we all experience frequently. When I snapped at her, I was overly tired, I hadn't listened closely to what she said, and I felt irritated at not being understood. I didn't face the situation with self-discipline and maturity, so I didn't respond effectively.

We must understand that bad moods are distortions of reality, and they often propel us into acting in uncustomary ways. When we act in unusual ways, oftentimes destructively, we feel a little crazy, and so do the people we're with. When we're discouraged, the world looks like a dangerous place. When we're angry, we want to hurt others the same way we've been hurt. When we're frightened, we want to retreat into safety.

But what are you to do if your moods seem to come and go at will? Perhaps your mate has threatened to schedule you for a visit to a psychologist if you don't do something to become the person he or she married! Here are a few mood-stabilizing tips that I explain in greater detail in my book *The Power of Emotional Decision Making:*

- Feeling guilty about your moods won't help. You are not trying to have these moods, you didn't will them into existence, and you cannot simply will them away. Be easy on yourself.

- Consider moods as symptoms of other problems. With the right mind-set, you can use your moods to help you discover what else might be bothering you. Perhaps your outer layer of irritability is hiding some deeper hurt. You may be unhappy about your job, marriage, or friendships.

- Use your moods as opportunities to heal problems. Rather than regret your darker moods, let them help you learn and grow.

- Learn to express deeper emotions in healthier ways. Find a friend who will listen to your concerns, write in a journal, and seek counseling. Sometimes we need a skilled professional to help us sort out what we're feeling and what to do about it.

- Learn to anticipate a certain mood coming on. Instead of settling into that particular mood, make a conscious choice about what you will do. Will you settle into the mood, or will you take some action instead? Activity wards off many moods!

Fortunately, moods are *not* reality. We really are not different people, but the same person with many facets. As we strive to become healthy, we must integrate all of our feelings, thoughts, and actions into one cohesive, functioning person.

Searching for Gold

We may have pushed parts of ourselves out of our awareness, but we may find gold in our shadow. Our shadow side and our moods may confound us and make us feel crazy, but they also contain the possibility for our transformation.

This may not be a particularly fun exercise, but try it anyway: Consider the traits you possess but don't like to think about. Then consider the traits in others that you recognize and dislike. Chances are the very character traits that drive you crazy in others are the ones you also possess and try to disown. As the folks in the 12-step tradition say, "If you spot it, you got it."

Consider the times you overreact to a situation. This is prime shadow territory. When someone or something drives you crazy, your shadow is probably getting hooked. Conversely, if you notice and admire a quality in someone else, it may be a quality that you have but that you've disavowed because of a false sense of modesty.

Another way to search for gold is to look for the things you find yourself doing by accident. You cannot simply keep your shadow side quiet forever. For example, you may tell yourself you really like someone and then find a hundred reasons for avoiding him. Or you may tell yourself you are really a generous person and then act completely the opposite. That's your shadow side at work.

Searching for gold in your shadow and moods can be tremendously exciting. Discovering unlikeable aspects of our personality can be challenging, but it can also be like discovering an old friend after years of absence. Exploring your shadow can...

- help you understand why you act certain ways
- help you ask for something you're not currently getting in your life
- help you work through unfinished feelings
- help you break through old patterns of behavior

Perhaps the most exciting aspect of exploring your shadow and moods is learning to express emotions in a healthier way. Embracing your anger can help you set healthier boundaries in your life. Embracing sadness can open up the possibility of grieving old losses and connecting to others. Exploring fear can help us better understand the realities of a frightening situation and discover new ways of being. Embracing joy can inspire us to live our dreams.

Exposing parts of your shadow can feel risky, but remember, it's all good. Whenever I become frightened about discovering parts of myself, I remind myself of a skit I saw years ago.

Criticizer: "You're really selfish sometimes."

Person: "Yes, I am. I've discovered that about myself and don't like it any more than you do."

Criticizer: "You tend to think too much of yourself too."

> Person: "Yes, that's also true, and you haven't seen the worst of
> me. Imagine what I'm like when I'm really full of my-
> self."
>
> Criticizer: "You really need to change that quality about
> yourself."
>
> Person: "You're absolutely right. I recognize my need to
> change, and I'm going to do it."

Can you see the value in embracing criticism? You don't have to own everything the criticizer is saying, but surely you can find at least a kernel of truth in it. By "trying it on," you're taking the wind out of your critic's sail as well as edging closer to your own weaknesses.

I'm not proposing we all set out to amplify our mistakes and moodiness, but simply to get a bit more comfortable with our shadow. Smiling at our mistakes can help us accept them and then allow God to do His transforming work. This is also a fabulous way of allowing others to be human with us.

Loved into Acceptance

We all struggle to accept various parts of our personality. In fact, this lack of acceptance, or the rejection of our various parts, is what makes us fragmented and a bit crazy. Our loving acceptance of ourselves and others is the critical key to healing.

Drs. Les and Leslie Parrott, in their book *Becoming Soul Mates,* offer a version of the German fairy tale Rapunzel. The Parrotts suggest this is a story of a beautiful girl who is imprisoned in a tower with an old witch who repeatedly tells her she is ugly. One day, Rapunzel gazes from the window of the tower and sees a prince standing below. In those famous words he cries, "Rapunzel, Rapunzel, let down your hair." She does so, and the prince braids her tresses into a ladder so he can rescue her.

> The implicit message of this fairy tale is simple but profound.
> Rapunzel's prison is really not the tower but her fear that

she is ugly and unlovable. The mirroring eyes of her prince, however, tell her that she is loved, and thus she is set free from the tyranny of her own imagined worthlessness.[1]

We have some awareness of our weaknesses, but we often try to push them away. We have memories of maltreatment by a harsh parent, grandparent, or critical caretaker. In an effort to survive, we try to banish these negative voices, usually unsuccessfully. We can relate with Rapunzel—we want to be beautiful and desirable, but we feel ugly and rejected.

Rapunzel is saved by the adoring prince. We too can be saved by those who would dare to accept us. Rather than splintering off our unpleasant shadow, we must bring it into the light of God's acceptance as well as the acceptance of others who care about us. We must be brave enough to fully own our darkest secrets and place them in the refiner's fire (Psalm 66:10; Isaiah 48:10; 1 Peter 1:7). Here in the heated crucible, our weaknesses become strengths.

The apostle Paul offers us another example of being loved into acceptance. Feeling completely accepted by Christ, Paul shared about his "thorn in the flesh." He reveals that he prayed three times that this weakness be taken from him. "But he [the Lord] said to me, 'My grace is sufficient for you, for my power is made perfect in weakness.' Therefore I will boast all the more gladly about my weakness, so that Christ's power may rest on me" (2 Corinthians 12:9).

Paul felt loved and accepted, so he was willing to accept and even boast about his weaknesses, which God used to illustrate His power. Paul learned to transcend his limitations, and we can do the same. Sensing God's incredible acceptance, we can accept ourselves and others. We can provide a safe place to ask for our needs to be met, and we can extend ourselves to meet the needs of others.

The Trauma of Transparency

Have you found a place where you are loved, faults and all? Have you experienced the freedom that comes with revealing your warts to accepting people? That is where we grow into the people God wants us to be.

Even with all this encouragement, you may still be afraid to expose all of your weaknesses. We have been trained to impress, impersonate, and put on a show since we were young. Rarely are we told to be exactly who we are. Rarely do we sit in a circle, hold hands, and share our deepest fears and greatest failures.

We can easily encourage others to be themselves while we hide behind a cloak of self-righteousness. We'd rather die than have others peek behind the scenes and see how we really are when no one is watching. Transparency can be traumatic.

However, if you want to be healthy and to rid yourself forever of those nagging feelings of craziness, you must stand up straight, cock your head forward, and tell the truth—at least to some people. You need to have some places where you don't dress to impress. You need some people who know everything about you and still love and accept you. This is scary stuff. It's always been scary stuff. Since the beginning of time we've been hesitant to share ourselves with others, though this is the only way of coming out of isolation and into relationship.

J. Grant Howard, in his book *The Trauma of Transparency*, explains that God created us to be transparent. He created Adam and Eve to be completely available for each other.

> The garden scene was unique in the annals of human history. God and man involved in totally open and honest communication with one another. Each saying what needed to be said—in the right way, at the right time, and for the right purpose. Here for the moment was that delicately balanced combination of truth and transparency that the world now struggles to understand and achieve.[2]

We all want to go back to the garden, but that's not possible. We want that level of transparency and honesty, but we've been struggling with openness ever since the Fall. In a world filled with distrust, we're cautious. Fearing being exposed as frauds, we put on our different faces. We act one way with friends, another with family, and perhaps yet another at the workplace. No wonder we feel schizophrenic.

But again, we're not as crazy as we think. We're all out to make a good impression. We all have certain images in our mind that we strive to emulate. The truth of the matter is, we are neither as good as we might think nor as bad as we might fear.

Getting Real

We're all feeling a bit crazy, yet thankfully, we're not as crazy as we think. Resolving our feelings of craziness requires work—getting real. Being real requires that our insides match our outsides. Our values and beliefs must match our behavior. This can be a tall order. You can't be completely congruent in every aspect of your life, but you can know yourself and have the courage to know when you're putting on an act and when you're being completely real.

What should I say to Madeline if she is putting up a front, as Hank suggests? How do I make her feel safe enough to reveal the depth of her pain and the incongruity of her actions? The burden falls largely on my shoulders—I must give her the space and comfort she needs to share with me what is really happening in her world. Accurate empathy is deceptively healing. If she feels that I understand the severity of her situation and acknowledge that we all act differently than we believe, perhaps she'll reveal more of her self to me.

Being real requires safety. Being real requires an environment where you won't be mocked or shamed into hiding your true qualities. Being real means looking around and realizing we're all in this boat together. Anything you've done, I've either done or imagined doing.

Being exactly who you are is OK. You're not as crazy as you think. We all have secrets, thoughts, and actions that embarrass us. We have parts of ourselves that we've pushed into our shadow, and we're all working at integrating them into our personality. That's what getting real is all about.

I've said before that I'm privileged to be allowed into the secret chambers of people's hearts. In my counseling office, people share their deepest fears, the longings they've told no one, and the harsh and painful realities of their lives. I'm always delighted to tell them this:

> You have these deep fears. You have years of hurt and pain, and your life has blemishes. You think these detract from the person you'd like to be, but in fact they don't detract at all. Like the Velveteen Rabbit, your missing buttons and frayed binding make you more real. You are much like everyone else who comes to see me, frightened that others will notice these blemishes.
>
> If you are to learn how to accept yourself, you must realize that we're all flawed. We all have missing buttons, stains, hurts, and insecurities. We can help each other by holding hands, looking unflinchingly into one another's eyes, and offering acceptance. You are loved for who you are, not for who you're striving to be.

Without fail, people let out a sigh of relief when they hear this. We're desperate to feel understood and accepted for who we are. We're anxious to hear that we're not as crazy as we think and that others have the same fears, hurts, wounds, and emotions we do. We want to fit in. Instead of hiding and trying to project an image of perfection, we would do well to let our blemishes show, as frightening as this is. When we do this, we give others permission to do the same. We invite others to be fully human. When we do this, we discover a powerful and healing truth: We're not as crazy as we think.

Epilogue:
Perfectly You

*Certain flaws are necessary for the whole. It would
seem strange if old friends lacked certain quirks.*

GOETHE

You're not as crazy as you think. Oh, I know you still have doubts. Your family tells you you're a quarter turn off. Your friends in counseling remind you that your behavior fits the criteria for XYZ personality disorder, according to the *American Psychiatric Association's Diagnostic Statistical Manual,* fourth edition. Nonetheless, I'm absolutely convinced you're not as crazy as you think.

How do I know this? My 34 years of counseling experience, working with thousands of people, gives me some authority on the matter. I hope hearing that from an authority gives you at least some relief.

Sometimes it surprises me how much time and attention we give to this issue of personality. How often (be honest!) do you leave a family get-together and talk about everyone in the family? How often do you come home from work and grouse about the mental fortitude of your boss or coworkers? How often do you secretly wonder about your own mental stability?

We all know the answer to these questions. We're all excessively preoccupied with the whole issue of personality traits. We're far too concerned with ourselves, when in reality, we're all a little bit nuts and would do well to get comfortable with that truth. It's time to stop taking ourselves so seriously!

I hope I've completely established that there are no perfect people. Thank goodness. No one has the corner on the market of normalcy. In fact, defining normalcy is next to impossible. Technically speaking, normal means average or typical, and who wants to be that? We're all a little bit nuts with plenty of quirks and idiosyncrasies, so we can all sit back and enjoy our abnormality.

Instead of fussing about normalcy or abnormality, we'd be better served capitalizing on our strengths. After all, we can build on our strengths much more easily than we can improve our weaknesses. The combination of weaknesses and strengths comprise this entity called *you*, and that is what I want you to embrace. Being perfect means being perfectly you!

For Your Review

Any good epilogue should remind you where we've been, and what exactly you should take away from this book. Here we go...

First of all, we can easily be swept into the eddy of worry by trying to define and adapt to this thing called *normal*. What is normal, anyway? Who gets to define these things? Normalcy is probably defined by a bunch of stuffed shirts, so I suggest we loosen up and broaden the definitions of normal and hereby grant that all readers of this book are normal or above.

Unfortunately, some people will be presumptuous enough to judge themselves normal and us crazy. Avoid these people, or at least be cautious with them. They insist that everyone should be just like them. If we give them a voice of authority, we'll always come up with the short end of the stick. Comparisons kill.

We spent an entire chapter talking about whether you even want to be normal. If you could wave a magic wand or change yourself into the perfect picture of normalcy, would you do it? I seriously hope not. This world needs variety. We would be a very bland and tepid group indeed if we melded ourselves together into a sea of monotony.

We also talked about our tendency to worry that people are talking about us. In fact, sometimes they do. You can be sure that the second you leave your family gathering, office party, or other engagement, you'll be the topic of conversation for a minute or two (if that long). You're not as crazy as you think and possibly not as popular. Sorry.

We spend too much energy trying to be like others. Sifting through the magazines at the checkout counter of the grocery store may be great entertainment, but it's not a good way to determine whether we're crazy. Celebrities will never help us determine whether some part of our personality needs attention.

As much as we strive to be ourselves, many of us get pulled into the current of sameness. Part of us wants to blend in and be just like others. You know the routine—shout to the world your individuality while you dress exactly like those in your peer group. There goes your individuality. Now you see me, now you don't.

We discussed how to deal effectively with secrets—the parts of our lives we keep hidden. Do we admit we have them? Why do we keep them? Should we reveal some? Why? How many? Some of us have a lot of secrets, and we feel a bit insecure about them. Others tell everything about themselves to the people sitting next to them on the bus or airplane. Generally speaking, it's best to find a balance between the two. Without a doubt, having a history, replete with issues causing embarrassment, makes you a bona fide member of the human race.

We spent a chapter talking about the killer of the human psyche—stress, which can lead to that all-too-common feeling of being on the brink of a nervous breakdown, whatever that is. We've all had our crises and felt as if one more molecule of stress would push us over some imaginary ledge. But thankfully, it's just stress, not some mental aberration. We're learning to live more effectively, trying a little harder to manage our stress so it doesn't manage us.

But what about the people who are ruled by their emotions—who suffer from emotional myopia? Some feel overwhelmed by feelings of sadness, anger, or hurt. Did we all agree that those people need some special psychological attention? No. We agreed that our emotions are wonderful, God-given tools to help us know what needs attention in our lives. We shouldn't be ruled by our emotions, but we don't want to be robots either. Again, balance is key.

We spent some time talking about our families. Ah, now here's where things got very interesting. Every family has its parade of unique people. Some have eccentrics, and others have flamboyant person-alities. Some have loners, and others have sufferers. Every family is completely unique, like a fingerprint in the vast conglomeration of society. In the midst of family chaos, we believe our family is certifi-ably nuts. Your family is probably comparable to many others in one way or another.

Finally, we talked about how to live together with our idiosyncrasies. When you're hooked for life with someone whom you consider too emotional, too uptight, too persnickety, too cranky, or whatever, what are you to do? You learn the dance of the porcupines. With healthy boundaries and a lot of practice, you'll do fine.

A Final Story

Now it's time for a final story to illustrate the importance of cut-ting yourself a huge amount of slack. The story portrays the truth that things (including people) are not exactly the way they appear. Beneath the surface, we're all a little bit nuts.

A while back, a middle-aged woman called asking for help with her marriage. With precise, measured speech, she described a very privileged life in California, where both she and her husband were professional people.

"What's the problem?" I asked.

"My husband has been hiding money, cheating on me, and being deceptive about the whole thing," Sandy said. Resentment oozed from her words.

"It's my second marriage, though," she continued, "and I'd really like to save it. I want my husband to come clean so we can get on with our lives."

"How do you know he's guilty of all that?" I questioned.

"Oh, I know all right. I've got paperwork proving he had an affair a few years ago. And the money can't be as tight as he makes out. He's lying about a lot of it."

I spent several sessions on the phone with her, becoming convinced that her husband was a philanderer and liar. The woman sounded like she was being victimized and was rightfully angry about it. After several hours of talking, we agreed it was time to talk to her husband, Phil. I made a phone call to him to discuss the matter.

Flabbergasted at the complaints, he rendered an entirely different story.

"She's always been paranoid, doctor," he said calmly. "Look, I'm a professional man and a Christian. I have no desire to cheat on her. As for the money, it's all right there in the checkbook. No hidden accounts. We've gone to counseling several times to talk about these things, and each time she quits because she doesn't like what she hears."

We agreed to talk again, with me being more than a little confused. Reality is stranger than fiction, or at least so it seemed with this couple.

I spent the next several weeks gathering information, trying to help them sort out the truth of their situation. I felt increasingly crazy, and I'm sure they did too. Each had a conspiracy theory going about the other, portraying the other as the villain and themselves as the victim.

Finally I decided there was no way and perhaps no reason to get to the bottom of things. Would it make any real difference? Phil and Sandy had a great deal of distrust to work through, but both wanted to end the years of acrimony and get a fresh start.

We agreed they would fly up to a Marriage Intensive, where I work with a couple intensively over several days. During their several days with me, we were able to sort some of their issues out, though parts were left up in the air. Sandy decided that though she still had a bit of uncertainty, she could find no real evidence of philandering, hidden bank accounts, or deception. Only bruised egos and years of distrust.

I discovered again what I've discovered thousands of times: We're all a little bit nuts, but we're not as crazy as we think. Both were able to find a degree of acceptance of the other, which was a wonderful starting place for healing.

Through a Different Lens

Of course it was gratifying to help Sandy and Phil sort through their differences. It was amazing to watch the years of distrust and resentment fall by the wayside. It was a pleasure to see them begin to communicate effectively rather than with innuendo, avoidance, and antagonism.

What made all the difference to this couple? They had to put down one lens and pick up another. They had to see each other and themselves through a different lens. They had to let go of a presumptuous attitude and take on an attitude of humility.

With hours of careful listening and cooperation, Sandy was able to see that Phil was not a cheating, deceptive man lacking any moral fiber, but an honest man. Phil was able to understand how Sandy could distrust him when he didn't share as openly as he might. He agreed to communicate more effectively.

Laying down one lens and picking up another can be more difficult than you might imagine. We become invested in the way we see things, so gaining a new point of view is nearly impossible. But that is what we need to do if we want to establish a more realistic concept of ourselves and other people.

Rather than seeing ourselves as deficient, lacking, and possibly even a bit crazy, we can zoom out and see ourselves from a larger point of view. From this larger, broader perspective, we see that we're not nearly as crazy as we think. We see that others aren't as crazy as we think either.

And what is that new point of view? How should we view ourselves?

This is where Scripture is wonderfully helpful. Let's review what the Bible has to say about how we are to view ourselves. Its truths can help us feel a lot more normal and a lot less crazy. The Scriptures are our final authority, and they clearly tell us that God made us the way we are, He loves us, and He has made a place for us. The only logical conclusion is this: The way to be perfect is to be perfectly you.

One Body, Many Parts

The Scriptures offer a powerful lens through which we can view one another. Rather than demanding we all see things exactly the same way or behave robotically with one another, Scripture encourages individuality. The apostle Paul informs us about an incredible truth: None of us are dispensable in the Scriptural economy. In an amazing passage of Scripture, Paul describes the family of God as a human body. Just as each part of the human body is critical for complete functioning, each of us is critical to the family of God.

> The human body has many parts, but the many parts make up one whole body. So it is with the body of Christ...But our bodies have many parts, and God has put each part just where he wants it. How strange a body would be if it had only one part! Yes, there are many parts, but one body (1 Corinthians 12:12,18-20 NLT).

Paul goes on to emphasize the importance of each individual part. The eye should never try to be an ear, and the ear should never try to be an eye. Each plays a vital role in the functioning of the body. Similarly, Paul points out the value of each member of the body of Christ. We all have differing gifts, and each is imperative to the full functioning of the body.

What does this say to us? We must always live within our gifting. We must be exactly who God has called us to be. Nothing more and certainly nothing less.

Who are you? What desires, gifts, and special concerns has God placed within you? How are you different from others? Your uniqueness is one aspect of your special gifting. The ways you are different from others may help reveal your unique gifting to the world. So rather than lamenting your individuality, consider your special gift to others.

Since We're Neighbors...

So we're a hodgepodge of people. We all have quirks and characteristics that make us unique and possibly a little bit strange to others. Still, we're not as crazy as we think, and since we're neighbors—and family and colleagues—we might as well be friends.

We're actually called to be more than friends. We're prone to be critical of anyone of different faith, color, beliefs, or appearance, but the Scriptures make a strong demand on us. A religious leader, seeking to test Jesus, asked him, "Who is my neighbor?" Jesus answers with a story.

> A Jewish man was traveling on a trip from Jerusalem to Jericho, and he was attacked by bandits. They stripped him of his clothes, beat him up, and left him half dead beside the road.
>
> By chance a priest came along. But when they saw him lying there, he crossed to the other side of the road and passed him by. A Temple assistant walked over and looked at him lying there, but he also passed by on the other side.
>
> Then a despised Samaritan came along, and when he saw the man, he felt compassion for him. Going over to him, the Samaritan soothed his wounds with olive oil and wine and bandaged them (Luke 10:30-34 NLT).

Jesus asks a piercing question: "Which of these three would you say was a neighbor to the man who was attacked by bandits?" Of course it was the one who showed mercy. Jesus calls us to take the high road: "Now go and do the same" (verses 36-37).

In her powerful book *Amazing Grace*, Kathleen Norris challenges us to tear down dividing walls.

The story of the good Samaritan seems as reckless and scary in its demands on the human heart as what God tells Moses on the mountaintop—do all that I have asked of you, get Pharaoh to release the people, come here and worship on this mountain, and only then will you know that I am your God.[1]

As I consider my life, filled to the brim with a wife, grown children, several siblings, two parents, numerous colleagues, employees, neighbors, and friends, I see a disjointed array of people. Some are rich, some poor. Some are Caucasian, some of color. Some are outgoing and friendly, others are introverted and quiet. Some are immensely likeable, and some aren't. All are children of God with a desperate need for compassion.

This book is primarily a declaration that we spend far too much time focusing on differences and far too little time focusing on similarities. Noticing differences, we spend too much time labeling, judging, and criticizing, and too little time holding hands, showing compassion, and valuing the unique contribution others make to our lives. What would we do, after all, if our old friends suddenly lacked their quirks?

Notes

Chapter 1—Crazy, Normal, or Something In Between?

1. Ralph Swindle, Kenneth Heller, Bernice Pescosolido, and Saeko Kikuzawa, "Responses to nervous breakdowns in America over a 40-year period: Mental health policy implications," *American Psychologist,* 55(7): 740-49.
2. David Sheehan, *The Anxiety Disease* (New York: Bantam Books, 1983), 35.

Chapter 2—Everyone Looks So Normal

1. Barbara Sher, *It's Only Too Late If You Don't Start Now* (New York: Random House, 1998), 146.
2. Reuters, "No second thoughts as Favre packs it in." Available online at www.abc.net .au/news/stories/2008/03/07/2182947.htm.
3. David Allyn, *I Can't Believe I Just Did That* (New York: Tarcher, 2004), 10.
4. J. Grant Howard, *The Trauma of Transparency* (Portland, OR: Multnomah Press, 1979), 41.

Chapter 3—Courageously Exploring Inner Space

1. M. Scott Peck, *The Road Less Traveled* (New York: Touchstone, 1978), 52-53.
2. Cheryl Richardson, *Take Time for Your Life* (New York: Broadway Books, 1998), 24.
3. Ibid., 25.
4. Joy Browne, *The Nine Fantasies That Will Ruin Your Life* (New York: Three Rivers Press, 1998), 22.
5. Gail Saltz, *Becoming Real* (New York: Riverhead Books, 2004), 16.

Chapter 4—You Really Want to Be Normal?

1. Peter Levitt, *Fingerpainting the Moon: Writing and Creativity as a Path to Freedom* (New York: Harmony Books, 2003), 26.

Chapter 5—We're All a Little Bit Nuts

1. Laura Schlessinger, *Bad Childhood, Good Life* (New York: HarperCollins, 2006), 23.
2. Ibid., 33.

Chapter 6—Everybody's Talkin' About Me

1. Parker Palmer, *A Hidden Wholeness* (New York: Jossey-Bass, 2004), 8-9.

236 ■ Normal People Do the Craziest Things

Chapter 7—Emotional Myopia

1. Barbara De Angelis, *How Did I Get Here?* (New York: St. Martin's Press, 2005), 47.
2. Melody Beattie, *Finding Your Way Home* (New York: HarperSanFrancisco, 1998), 181.

Chapter 8—If You Only Knew

1. Palmer, *A Hidden Wholeness,* 16.
2. Irwin Kula, *Yearnings* (New York: Hyperion, 2006), 26.

Chapter 9—But My Family *Is* Certifiably Nuts

1. Harriet Lerner, *The Dance of Anger* (New York: HarperCollins, 1997), 11.
2. Melody Beattie, *Codependent No More* (Center City, MN: Hazelden, 1987), 113.
3. Steven Farmer, *Adult Children of Abusive Parents* (New York: Ballantine Books, 1989), 151.
4. Virginia Satir, *Conjoint Family Therapy* (New York: Science and Behavior Books, 1983).
5. Harriet Lerner, *The Dance of Deception* (New York: HarperCollins, 1993), 89.
6. Schlessinger, *Bad Childhood, Good Life,* 23.

Chapter 10—Overwhelmed, Under Slept, and a Little Bit Tense

1. Adapted from Melinda Smith, Ellen Jaffe-Gill, and Jeanne Segal, "Understanding Stress: Signs, Symptoms, Causes, and Effects," HelpGuide.org. Available online at www.helpguide.org/mental/stress_signs.htm.
2. Edward Hallowell, *CrazyBusy* (New York: Ballantine Books, 2006), 4.
3. Sarah Susanka, *The Not So Big Life* (New York: Random House, 2007), 69.
4. Cecile Andrews, *Slow Is Beautiful* (Gabriola Island, BC: New Society Publishers, 2006), 180.

Chapter 11—Dance of the Porcupines

1. John Bradshaw, *Healing the Shame That Binds You* (Deerfield Beach, FL: Health Communications, 1988), 91.
2. Sue Patton Thoele, *The Courage to Be Yourself* (New York: MJB Books, 1988), 29.
3. Rosamund Stone Zander and Benjamin Zander, *The Art of Possibility* (New York: Penguin Books, 2002), 90.
4. Michael Gurian, *Love's Journey* (Boston: Shambhala Publishing, 1995), 150.
5. Linda Waite and Maggie Gallagher, *The Case for Marriage* (Toronto: Interim Publishing, 1999).

Chapter 12—Now You See Me, Now You Don't

1. Les Parrott and Leslie Parrott, *Becoming Soul Mates* (Grand Rapids: Zondervan, 1995), 65.
2. Howard, *The Trauma of Transparency,* 22-23.

Epilogue—Perfectly You

1. Kathleen Norris, *Amazing Grace* (New York: Riverhead Books, 1998), 354.

Marriage Intensives

Dr. David Hawkins has developed a unique and powerful ministry to couples who need more than weekly counseling. In a waterfront cottage on beautiful Puget Sound in the Pacific Northwest, Dr. Hawkins works with one couple at a time in Marriage Intensives over three days, breaking unhealthy patterns of conflict while acquiring new, powerful skills that can empower husbands and wives to restore their marriage to the love they once knew.

If you feel stuck in a relationship fraught with conflict and want to make positive changes working with Dr. Hawkins individually or as a couple, please contact him at 360.490.5446 or learn more about his Marriage Intensives at www.YourRelationshipDoctor.com.

Call Dr. Hawkins for professional phone consultations, or schedule him and his wife, Christie, for your next speaking engagement or marriage retreat.

■ ■ ■ ■

The Marriage Recovery Center

All couples experience instability and turmoil at times, but some experience severe crises and need special expertise. Dr. Hawkins, "The Relationship Doctor," opened the Marriage Recovery Center in 2006 to help couples in severe distress. With more than 30 years of clinical experience, Dr. Hawkins will help you and your mate recover from chronic conflict, resentment, and detachment. He will empower you and your mate to regain lost love and affection and restore your relationship to healthy functioning. To learn more about the Marriage Recovery Center, call Dr. Hawkins at 360.490.5446 or visit his website at www.YourRelationshipDoctor@yahoo.com.

Other Great Harvest House Books by Dr. David Hawkins

(To read sample chapters, visit www.harvesthousepublishers.com.)

WHEN PLEASING OTHERS IS HURTING YOU

When you begin to forfeit your own God-given calling and identity in an unhealthy desire to please others, you move from servanthood to codependency. This helpful guide can get you back on track.

DEALING WITH THE CRAZYMAKERS IN YOUR LIFE

People who live in chaos and shrug off responsibility can drive you crazy. If you are caught up in a disordered person's life, Dr. Hawkins helps you set boundaries, confront the behavior, and find peace.

NINE CRITICAL MISTAKES MOST COUPLES MAKE

Dr. Hawkins shows that complex relational problems usually spring from nine destructive habits couples fall into, and he offers practical suggestions for changing the way you and your spouse relate to each other.

WHEN THE MAN IN YOUR LIFE CAN'T COMMIT

With empathy and insight, Dr. Hawkins uncovers the telltale signs of commitment failure, why the problem exists, and how you can respond to create a life with the commitment-phobic man you love.

ARE YOU REALLY READY FOR LOVE?

As a single, you are faced with a challenge: When love comes your way, will you be ready? Dr. Hawkins encourages you to spend less energy looking for the perfect mate and more energy becoming a person who can enter wholeheartedly into intimate relationships.

HOW TO GET YOUR HUSBAND'S ATTENTION

She says one thing, but he hears something entirely different. What can you do to bridge the communication gap? This inspiring guide provides straightforward answers and practical solutions to encourage and motivate you to press through to the ultimate goal: greater intimacy in marriage.

THE POWER OF EMOTIONAL DECISION MAKING

"Energy in motion"—that's how Dr. Hawkins describes emotions. He shows how emotions can help you discern what is most important to you, determine what is missing in your life, and discover how God is leading you in new directions.

10 Lifesavers for Every Couple

Dr. Hawkins shows that times of relational stress are predictable and manageable. They can even lead to positive changes and renewed growth. Packed with biblical wisdom and practical information, this helpful manual affirms the value of marriage and empowers you to grow through your time of crisis.

Breaking Everyday Addictions

Addiction is a rapidly growing problem among Christians and non-Christians alike. Even socially acceptable behaviors, such as shopping, eating, working, playing, and exercising, can quietly take over and ruin your life. This enlightening exposé provides the tools you need to allow the healing power of Christ to permeate your life.

Wood Eaters

Written by Jill Eggleton

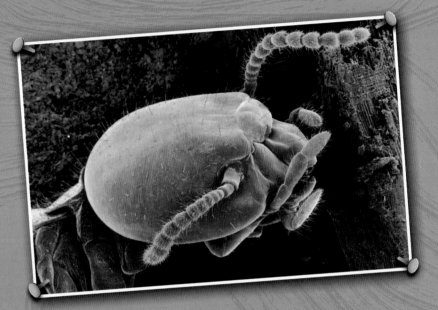

Contents

Invisible Pests 2
Termites 4
   Subterranean Termites 7
   Wood-dwelling Termites 8
   Termite Colonies 10
Woodworms 12
Wood-eating Fungi 14
Watch Out for Wood Eaters! 16
Index 17

Invisible Pests

Wood eaters are pests that are hard to find. They may eat away at wood for years and years and are only noticed when a wall collapses or a mound of sawdust appears on the ground.

Wood eaters, like termites, woodworms and wood-eating fungi, can be very destructive.

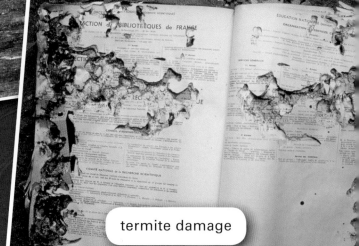

woodworm

termite damage

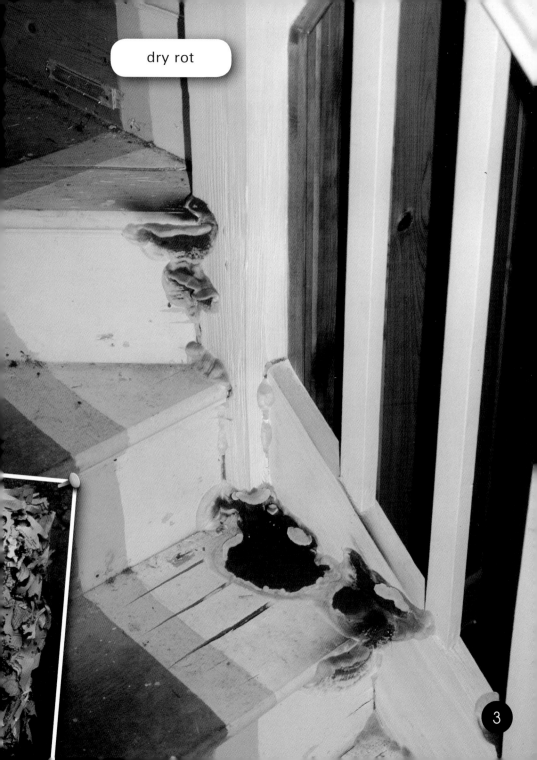

dry rot

3

Termites

Termites, or white ants as they are often called, are not really ants at all. They are closely related to cockroaches and just as old.

Termites date back to at least 100 million years ago, when there were no flowering plants, bees, birds or butterflies.

There are at least 2000 different types of termites. The termites that eat houses are wood-dwelling termites and subterranean termites.

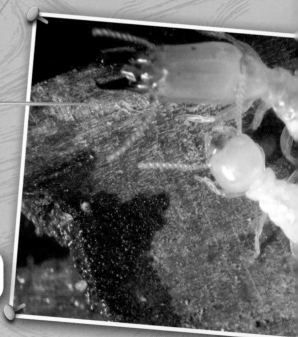

The cockroach is a relative of the termite.

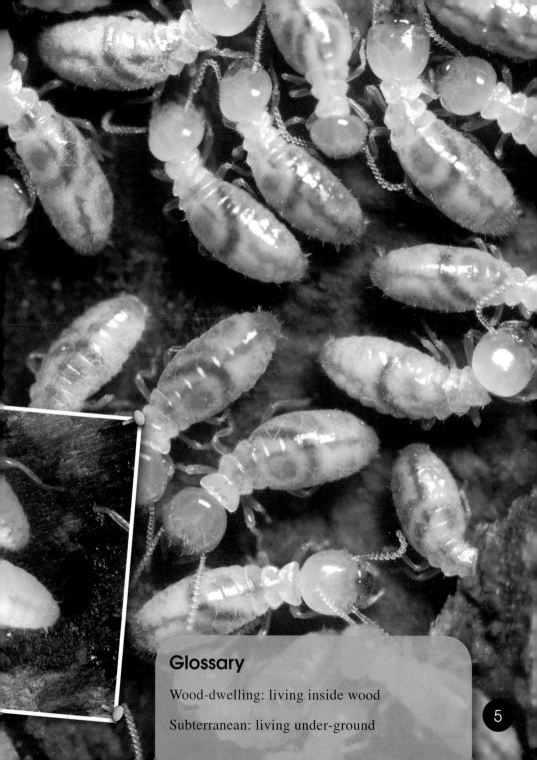

Glossary

Wood-dwelling: living inside wood

Subterranean: living under-ground

Termites live in communities like ants, with kings, queens, workers and soldiers. Their nests are called colonies. Each colony can have up to two million termites in it. Sometimes there will even be more than one queen.

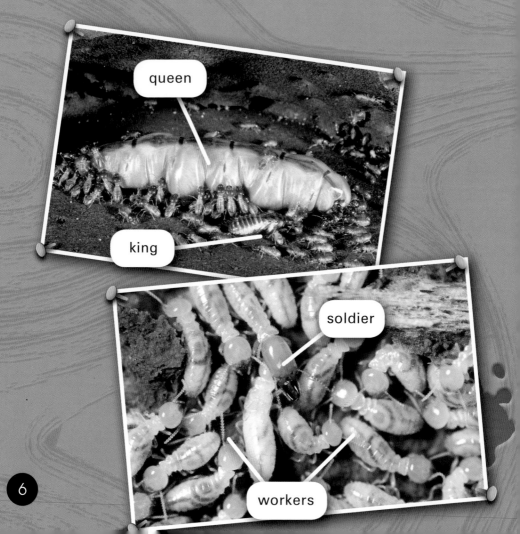

queen

king

soldier

workers

subterranean Termites

A colony of subterranean termites may be as deep as six metres below the soil surface. They travel through mud tubes to reach their food sources.

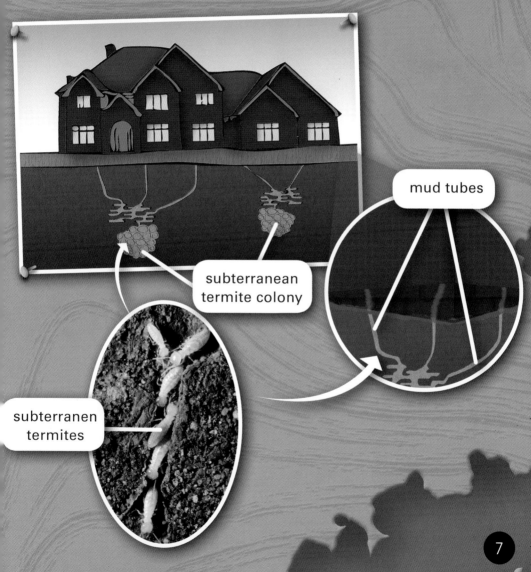

mud tubes

subterranean termite colony

subterranen termites

Wood-dwelling Termites

Wood-dwelling termites live inside the wood. They build bigger and bigger rooms for themselves as they eat.

They make small holes from their rooms to the outside world. Then they push their droppings out.

Small heaps of dung are a sign that wood-eating termites are in the wood, eating away.

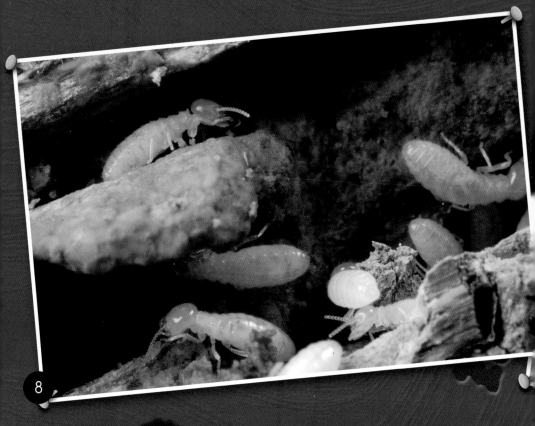

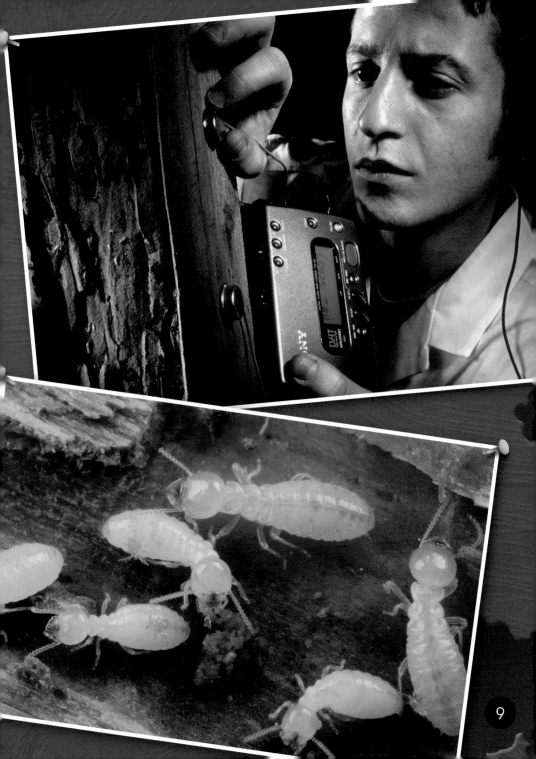

Termite Colonies

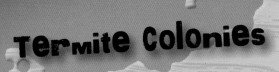

Termites cannot survive alone. They need their colony to protect them.

All termites work as one group. Each member of the group has a different job to do.

The queen termite lays the eggs. The workers, who are blind and wingless, gather the food. The soldiers provide protection with their large pincers.

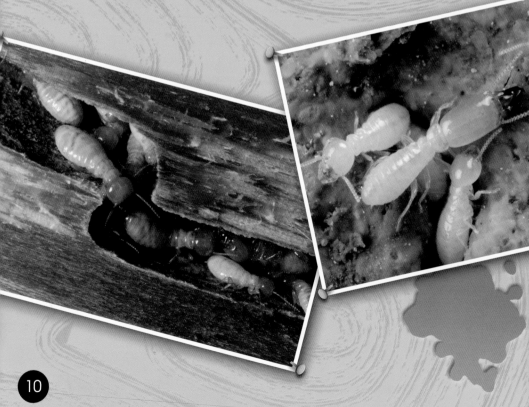

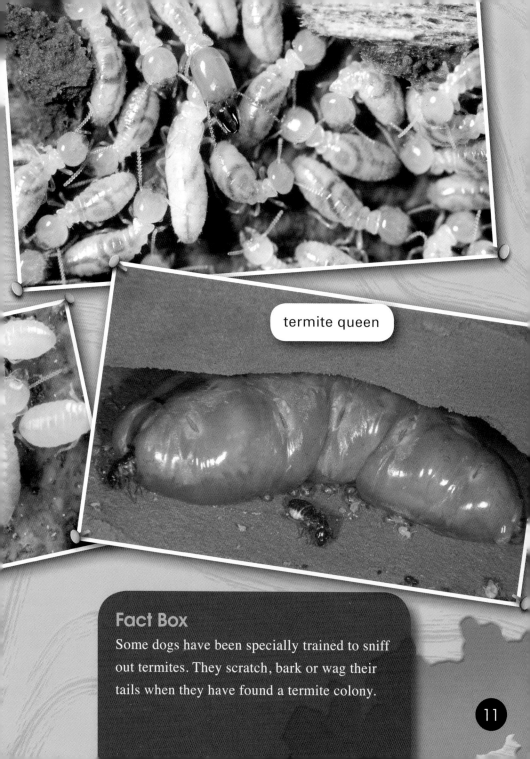

termite queen

Fact Box

Some dogs have been specially trained to sniff out termites. They scratch, bark or wag their tails when they have found a termite colony.

WoodWorms

Woodworms are soft and curved, with tiny legs. They are the worm stage of the furniture beetle. The adult beetles talk to each other by banging their bodies against the wood.

Woodworms can be found in dead and fallen timber. They attack window and door frames and wooden posts. They live by eating the wood.

Woodworms have become real pests in houses, planes and boats.

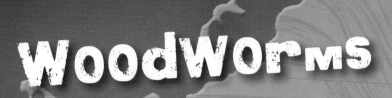

furniture beetle

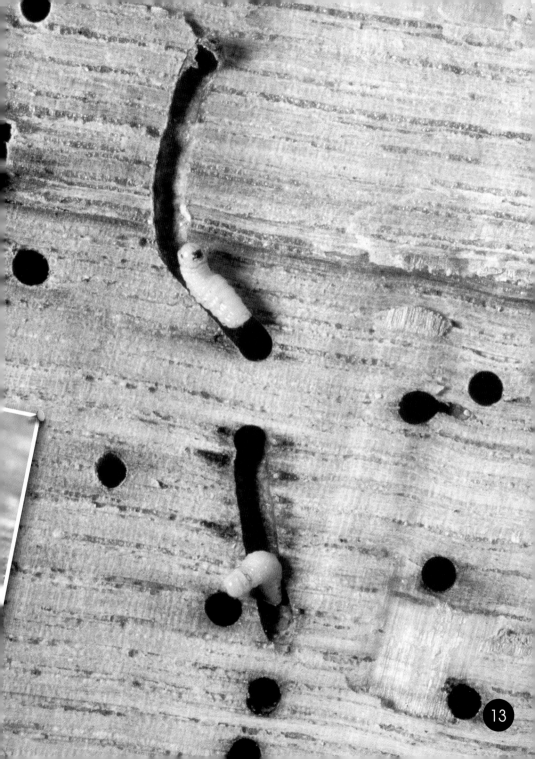

13

Wood-eating Fungi

Fungi are plants like mushrooms. They have to get food from green, growing plants or dead matter. Some fungi attack wood in houses when the wood is moist.

Dry rot in timber is caused by a fungus. Dry rot is actually wet. It looks like a white, thread-like tentacle and weaves through the wet wood, making it brittle.

These tentacles also carry water so the fungus can travel through dry wood, too. Dry rot destroys the dry wood as it goes. If wood with dry rot is pushed, it will fall apart.

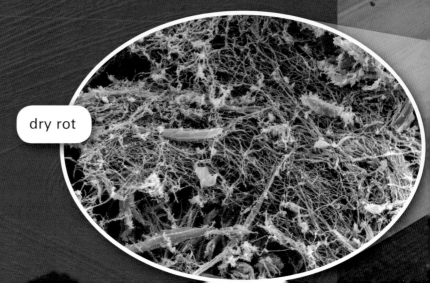

dry rot

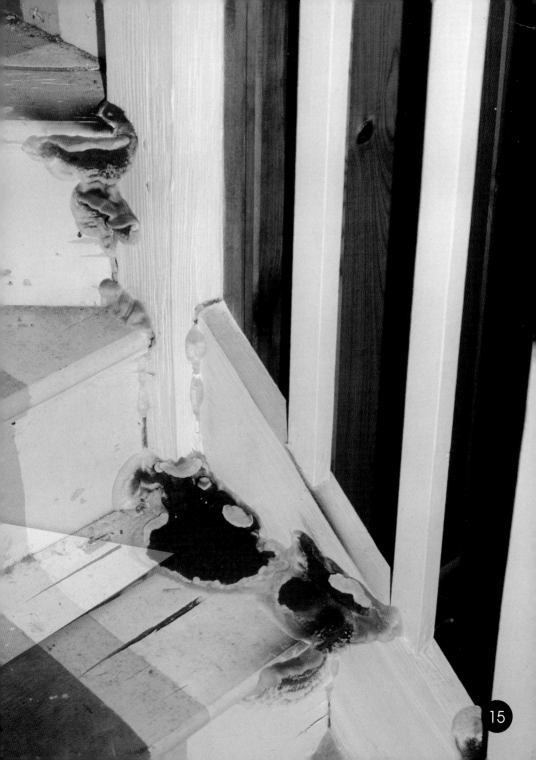

Watch Out for Wood Eaters!

woodworms

dry rot

wood-dwelling termites

subterranean termites

Index

cockroach   4

dry rot   14, 16

furniture beetle   12

mud tubes   7

pests   2, 12

subterranean termite 4, 7, 16

termite

    colony   6, 7, 10

    king   6

    queen   6, 10

    soldier   6, 10

    worker   6, 10

Reports

Wood Eaters is a Report.

A report has a topic:

Wood Eaters

A report has headings:

Wood-dwelling Termites

Wood-eating Fungi

Some information is put under headings.

> **Termites**
> _____
>
> - Termites live in nests called colonies.
> - There are kings, queens, workers and soldiers.

Information can be shown in other ways.
This report has ...

Labels   Photographs   Diagrams   Fact Box

Cross-section Diagram

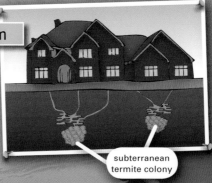

subterranean termite colony

Guide Notes

Title: **Wood Eaters**

Stage: Fluency

Text Form: Informational Report

Approach: Guided Reading

Processes: Thinking Critically, Exploring Language, Processing Information

Written and Visual Focus: Contents Page, Glossary, Labels, Cross-section Diagram, Fact Box, Index

THINKING CRITICALLY
(sample questions)

Before Reading – Establishing Prior Knowledge
- What do you know about animals and plants that eat wood?

Visualising the Text Content
- What might you expect to see in this book?
- What form of writing do you think will be used by the author?

Look at the contents page and index. Encourage the students to think about the information and make predictions about the text content.

After Reading – Interpreting the Text
- Do you think wood eaters are a good thing or not? Why do you think that?
- Why do you think termites need to live in colonies?
- What do you think could be some disadvantages of having to live under the ground? Why do you think that?
- What do you think could happen to a home if dry rot lived there?
- Do you think wood eaters are a good thing or not? Why do you think that?
- What do you know about animals and plants that eat wood that you did not know before?
- What in the book helped you to understand the information?
- What questions do you have after reading the text?

EXPLORING LANGUAGE

Terminology
Photograph credits, index, contents page, imprint information, ISBN number